LIVING WITH LEUKAEMIA

and related disorders

Dr Pam McGrath

HILL OF CONTENT
MELBOURNE

First published in Australia 2001
by Hill of Content Publishing Pty Ltd
86 Bourke Street, Melbourne 3000
Tel: 03 9662 2282
Fax: 03 9662 2527
Email: hocpub@collinsbooks.com.au

Cover design: Deb Snibson Modern Art Production Group
Typeset by Midland Typesetters, Maryborough
Printed by Australian Print Group, Maryborough

National Library of Australia cataloguing-in-publication data:

McGrath, Pam.
Living with leukaemia : and related disorders.

ISB 085572 317 3.

1. Leukaemia – Popular works. 2. Leukaemia – Patients. I. Title.

616.99419

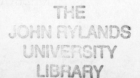

DEDICATION

This book is dedicated, with sincere appreciation, to all of those inspiring people who have so generously shared their stories with me during such a difficult time in their lives. It is my sincerest wish that this book goes some way to doing justice to your remarkable stories. The great privilege of working in this area is that I have constantly been witness to the power, strength and resilience of the human spirit.

ACKNOWLEDGMENTS

I would like to express my sincere appreciation to Dr Thomas Koilparampil, Director, Regional Cancer Centre, Trivandrum, India, for proof reading and reviewing the clinical appendices of this book. It is a great honour to have such an excellent clinician and international leader in oncology affirm the reliability of the translation of the medical information to lay language.

I would also like to sincerely thank my daughter Emma for making the time during her very busy life to proof read the manuscript for this book.

Finally, I would like to acknowledge with appreciation and love the support and enthusiasm I have received for this project from my four lovely daughters, Amy, Emma, Zoë and Bo. You are a constant reminder to me that, with courage and determination, individuals can deal successfully with the many difficulties associated with the challenge of *Living with Leukaemia*. Thank you for your love and your inspiration.

CONTENTS

Chapter 1

INTRODUCTION

If you have this book in your hand and are reading these words, the odds are that either you or a loved one have in some way been touched by the life-altering experience of being diagnosed with leukaemia or an associated haematological malignancy. If so, then read on, this book is written especially for you. The aim of the book is to provide the basic information you need to survive this experience, written in a way that is easy for you to understand.

The background to the book

The content of *Living with Leukaemia* has been written from years of experience working with and talking to individuals and their families who are coping with a diagnosis of leukaemia or a related disorder. Although not designed to be an academic book, all of the discussion will be informed by extensively researched information on the topic. For years I have been conducting research projects on the psycho-social aspects of haematological malignancies along the full continuum of life from infancy to adulthood. My work has been driven by an open-ended qualitative perspective that simply seeks to listen and record. Such research is not driven by the assumptions and questionnaires of experts but by a desire to listen to the insights of those who have first-hand experience with these illnesses and treatments. So much of the information in this book has been gained from you, my reader, and I am only now returning it to you, with thanks.

A difficult journey

Living with Leukaemia makes no apology for stating that this is a difficult journey. This will certainly not be a revelation for those presently coping with these disorders. An assumption underpinning this book is that it is only when the full extent of the difficulties involved in this journey are known that the provision of appropriate services will be possible. Only then will all of those involved in providing care and support have the understanding to respond appropriately and with compassion.

The central message

The central message of this book is that, because dealing with a haematological disorder can be one of life's difficult challenges, it may help if you re-establish your sense of normality in relation to others going through the same journey. All too often people do not have the chance to share experiences with others in similar situations, to be inspired by those who have really 'been there, done that'. For those without these contacts, this is your own personal conversation with many many others who have had to cope with similar life challenges. This book will always be there for you when you feel the need to absorb the strength offered by the collective wisdom and insights of others who have been your way. The hope and expectation in writing the book is that, as you see yourself or your family reflected in the stories of others, you will gain strength from the knowledge that you are not alone in what can seem a 'reality-altering' experience.

A secondary hope and expectation in writing this book is that it will also be read by the many health and allied health care professionals who care for you. Much of the medical drama in relation to haematological malignancies is acted out in the very structured and busy environment of the hospital ward. All involved have busy schedules and, although sympathetic to the needs and concerns of patients and their families, will not have the space to share your experience in any depth. Hospital roles are structured, with each person knowing their duties and appropriate ways of acting. Typically, patients and their families try to present their best and can also feel somewhat intimidated by the hospital routine. In short, it is not an environment conducive to finding out what is happening in the lives of others. It is thus hoped that the story provided by this book will provide insights into the difficulties faced by patients and their families which will go some way to informing necessary support services both in the hospital and in the community.

Learning a 'new language'

This is a highly technical area of health care where professionals are known to 'talk another language' of complicated terminology and sophisticated ideas. It is usual for individuals to feel overwhelmed and disoriented whilst they are learning 'the language'. Unfortunately, all too often, important decisions have to be made quickly and without warning during the steep learning curve of initiation into the world of haematology. Thus, this book is written to assist you to access as easily as possible the information you need, at the pace that you want to absorb it.

It is not assumed that you will want to read, or indeed know about, everything to do with these diagnostic groups. Indeed, it is now well documented that individuals will differ widely in what they want to know. Some people will thrive on gathering as much information as possible and will be energised by knowledge about their situation. Others require only sufficient information to cope with their present challenges and will recoil from being overloaded with too many facts. The chapters are separated into specific areas of interest and are organised under headings which will allow you to pick and choose what you want to know. For those who seek more detailed knowledge than the book can provide, there will be references in the appendices for further in-depth readings.

Although titled *Living with Leukaemia*, the book covers a wide range of diagnostic groups, including leukaemia and related blood disorders such as myelomas and lymphomas. It is most likely that each reader will be scanning the book for information on one particular diagnostic group. However, much of the information is generic and has relevance for all who must cope with these disorders. Indeed, one of the reasons for writing this book is that it has become obvious through research that there is a great similarity in the experience of those who have to cope with this group of disorders as compared to other areas of oncology or chronic illnesses. This is, perhaps, because of the long treatment protocols and the high-tech treatments. Hence there will be many times throughout this book when a generic term will be needed to indicate that reference is being made to the full range of diagnostic groups. At such times the term 'haematological malignancies' will be used. Although somewhat cumbersome, it is the correct and all-inclusive term.

The whole story

Living with Leukaemia does not, however, focus narrowly on the physical body. An important assumption underlying the content of this book is that the challenge of coping with a haematological malignancy will make demands on the emotional, social, financial and spiritual resources of the diagnosed individual and their families. It is now understood that individuals can be greatly assisted by information that provides insights into the shared human experience of this journey. The simple message underpinning the material offered in this book is that if you can hear some of the experiences of others you will come to feel much more confident about your own ability to cope. Without this information it is easy for individuals to feel isolated and alone in dealing with the challenges presented. Information about what others go through and how they cope can go some way to normalising your experience.

Concluding comment

It has always been my experience in interviewing people that, in the midst of relating their own very profound problems, they unself-consciously comment with compassion on the plight of others. In spite of the profound difficulties people face, they are only too ready to look into the lives of others and compassionately think 'there but for the grace of God go I'. It is humbling and awe-inspiring to be witness to such strength of the human spirit in the face of such adversity. It is my most genuine wish that this book does justice to the sheer difficulty of your journey and, in so doing, helps you and those who care for you to realise that *Living with Leukaemia* is a feat that displays quite considerable courage and tenacity.

Chapter 2

EARLY DAYS

Most stories start out with a gentle plot that gradually builds to the point of a significant event. The author provides an endless stream of hints or clues that prepares the reader for the possibility of a poignant happening. With the exception of a few chronic conditions, such a luxury is not afforded in relating the story of haematological malignancies because, as is now well known, perhaps the most difficult and dramatic time is at the very beginning, at the point of diagnosis.

The point of diagnosis

Many of the symptoms of haematological malignancies are fairly common complaints such as tiredness, bruising, or flu-like symptoms. Consequently, it is quite common to hear that patients, who will have an intuitive feeling that they have something more than a common virus, may have to consult many doctors or return many times to their own doctor before they can obtain a satisfactory diagnosis. Consequently, for some, receiving the diagnosis can partly be a relief as the patient at last has a disease label that confirms their intuitive sense. The label allows the individual to gain some insights as to what is happening to their body and thus to escape from the confusion of the unknown and be in the position to begin to build an appropriate response.

Others will not have had a lead-up time. The diagnosis may have been made as a result of blood tests from a routine check-up or during the early stage of the disease when the symptoms appear most unremarkable and certainly not associated with serious illness.

It is common for such patients to be left with a sense of disbelief and to require some time to come to terms with the reality of the information they are given.

The period following the point at which a person receives the diagnosis is now labelled an 'existential crisis' because receiving such news usually sends the individual into a state of shock. Individuals can feel a sense of emotional numbness as they start to process what they have been told. Physical symptoms of distress such as stomach upsets or inability to sleep can accompany this state. It is not unusual for individuals to feel somewhat distant from reality, as if they are unable to connect with others or the situation they are in. Many will have problems focusing on tasks or will find it hard to listen to and process information. Some will begin to confront directly the implications of the information they have been given and others will operate under degrees of denial, gradually assimilating the reality at an emotional pace suitable to their needs. Some will turn immediately for comfort to loved ones or friends and will seek the emotional release of sharing their feelings with those they are close to. Others will want lots of personal space to process the information on their own.

It will not only be the patient who experiences the shock but many within the intimate network of relationships. Particularly vulnerable in this regard are the parents of children diagnosed with such a condition. Receiving such news is considered to be one of the greatest hardships that a parent can face. Similarly, the news that a partner has been diagnosed, no matter how new or long term the relationship, can be a severe blow that will need time to come to terms with. However, this is not an area where generalisations can be made about the significance or implication of any diagnosis. For each person within the intimate circle the impact will depend on their own unique relationship and history to the person with the condition.

The rush to start treatment

Once diagnosed, however, the situation quickly changes. There is now a great deal that can be done to treat haematological malignancies.

Indeed, this is one of the most significant areas of success in cancer treatments. For example, childhood acute lymphoblastic leukaemia, a disease that was quickly lethal only two decades ago, now has a seventy to eighty per cent cure rate. A key factor in the success of treating such conditions is to start treatment immediately following diagnosis. Consequently, with the exception of a few chronic conditions, there is usually a strong urgency to start treatments for haematological malignancies immediately. Unfortunately, this means for many that treatment decisions will have to be made during the time when they are coping with the shock of diagnosis.

As most treatments for haematological malignancies require specialist care that is only available in a major metropolitan hospital, the majority of patients will have to travel. This process of having to leave the comfort of your own home to travel to a metropolitan hospital for specialist care is referred to as relocation for treatment.

The experience of relocation

Leaving immediately

The majority of people who have to relocate usually receive very little time between being told by their doctor that they possibly have a haematological disorder and having to make arrangements to travel to the metropolitan treatment centre.

As many of the tests for these sets of diseases require 'hi-tech' equipment and specialist understanding, the setting for confirming the diagnosis is usually the metropolitan centre. Thus, at the point of referral, although patients usually have some understanding of the possible diagnosis, they typically relocate with a high level of uncertainty about what is ahead of them. It is not unusual for patients to leave home with the expectation that they are only coming to the city for a few days of diagnostic testing and find they have to stay for many months for treatment.

At the point of departure, most people are in shock from hearing the possible diagnoses, are unsure of how long they will be away and have very little time to organise home and family before leaving. Consequently, many people arrive in the metropolitan centre with only a few possessions, with little idea of how long or where they are going to stay and with household arrangements at home left incomplete. Those that have been through the experience report that they do not have a clear enough 'head space' to be able to think logically about what to bring. Many who are used to coping well with life's demands are surprised at their confused state during this time.

At such a time family and friends can be of considerable assistance. Those who are fortunate enough to have such support report on the importance to them of the practical assistance provided by their loved ones. The assistance of friends or neighbours who come in to help organise children left behind, defrost the fridge, feed the pets, cut the grass or redirect the mail is deeply appreciated.

Not everyone has such support and these people have to cope under the added stress of knowing that so much is left undone at home. The suggestion has often been made to me that this is an important area where health care or community organisations could provide families with much needed support. Volunteers could make a real difference in this area if they undertook the responsibility of carrying out these tasks for families who need such support. Also, written check lists of items for packing and accommodation and support organisations that are available for families in the metropolitan area, provided at the point of referral, would assist in reducing the level of confusion experienced.

Putting life on hold

This is a time when individuals talk about having to 'put life on hold'. All of the normal experiences are suspended. Alternative arrangements have to be made for caring for family members, education, work and community activities. For many families this can mean major decisions have to be made, such as leaving work or education, that require significant readjustments in life.

Support from others can make an important difference. Employers who are sympathetic and send clear messages to individuals that their position will be kept open and their future employment is assured make a great difference. Indeed, many employers go to great lengths for their staff, some even become involved in fund-raising to assist families to cope. Sadly, there is a wide continuum of reactions from employers and not all respond with enlightened compassion to the plight of their employees. Particularly vulnerable individuals will be those who are self-employed. Unless their business is large enough for a person to delegate responsibility to another member of the firm, the self-employed, when confronted with illness, will have to cope with the quite considerable pressure of trying to maintain their business *in absentia*. Understandably, there are real difficulties for those working in independent, high maintenance occupations, such as farmers.

Educational activities can also be interrupted. Families often have to make difficult decisions about removing children from school in order to keep their family together. Where the protocols extend for over two years, as in some forms of leukaemia, the implications are great and the decisions challenging. There are special considerations for families with young children and these will be dealt with later.

Somewhere to stay

In the haste of making speedy arrangements for somewhere to stay, people often accept the offer to stay with relatives. At times this works out very well and the relatives are not only able to provide accommodation, but sometimes considerable practical and emotional support as well. There is, however, the potential for such arrangements to give rise to strained relationships. Often families who are thrown into close contact during such times of crisis, even with the best of good will, can experience considerable tension. As arrangements are made *ad hoc* they are not necessarily suitable in terms of nearness to the hospital or adequate space to accommodate everyone comfortably. This can be a particularly difficult situation in the case of young families where parents are trying to flex around the needs and demands of children. Such impromptu arrangements can be difficult to sustain.

Increasingly within the health care system there is becoming an awareness of the plight of relocated families. Most hospitals now have some form of accommodation available. There are also examples of leading community organisations providing excellent accommodation and support facilities. For example, a leading national organisation, the Leukaemia Foundation of Australia (LFA), has pioneered purpose-built accommodation centres for families. In Queensland, the LFA backs up the accommodation with a wide range of practical support services such as hospital transport, assistance with shopping, social activities, support counsellors, educational programs, a grief program and follow-up after returning home. If you are fortunate enough to access such accommodation services this will go a long way to reducing the stress for you. Not only will you have the privacy of your own unit to retreat to, but there will be practical assistance with such activities as transport to the hospital and shopping. You will be able to, at your own pace, meet others in a similar situation and will be provided with the opportunity to access educational programs and counselling if you wish. Unfortunately, such resources are not widely available and most families still have to depend on the resources within their own networks.

The alien world of the metropolitan city

Finding appropriate accommodation, however, is only part of the story. Many individuals, especially those who have never been to the city before, find the adjustment to metropolitan life daunting. At a time when individuals and their families are coping with the news of the diagnosis and the demands of initial treatment they must also learn to negotiate all the novel experiences of city living. Navigating the complex transport system of a large metro-politan centre can be frightening, especially if your previous experience has only been that of a small country town. For many, finding their way around the large shopping complexes, so common in the city, is another obstacle to be overcome. The simple task of grocery shopping can be stressful, for it entails understanding the transport system and the practical difficulty of physically carrying the goods home on public transport. This is particularly difficult if you are not well or you are a parent with a sick child.

This is an important area where the support of family and friends can make a significant difference, as there are many practical things others can do. Not everyone has such support, however, especially in a setting away from the comfort of his or her own home. Consequently, health and allied health care professionals need to be mindful of the enormous practical challenges of relocation and take proactive steps to ensure that individuals so affected have appropriate backup resources.

The brave new world of the metropolitan hospital

Not only is there an adjustment to be made to a new city environment, patients and their families have to learn to deal with the alien world of the 'hi-tech' metropolitan hospital for a disease that many know very little about. Many people can experience a form of culture shock where they must learn a new language and function in a world very different to anything they have previously known.

The language of haematology is complicated and is driven by a highly specialised area of medicine. To begin to make sense of the hospital environment the individual will need to absorb a wide range of concepts. Many will initially feel quite overwhelmed by the terminology. Entangled on the emotional roller-coaster of adjustment to diagnosis and treatment, the individual may not necessarily be in a receptive space. Suffice here to note that the requirement to speak this language is another challenge that is presented at a time when many individuals feel they already have too much to deal with. Fortunately, most do rise to the occasion and many eventually become more knowledgeable in this area than the health professionals they will eventually deal with when they return home. The next chapter will begin to outline the different styles of processing information and the appendices will provide, in easy to access format, the essentials of this language.

Not only will there be a battery of hi-tech procedures involved in diagnosing these illnesses but once the diagnostic group, staging and level of risk is known there will be innumerable tests needed to initiate and monitor treatment. For many individuals, this can be an invasive experience at a time that they are only just coping with all the other adjustments they have to make. Hospital strategies that try to minimise the sheer number of tests and reduce the number of personnel involved during this stage go some way to helping individuals cope. Modern treating hospitals can be complex places with a vast array of diagnostic centres, outpatient and in-patient treatment facilities. Even the experienced hospital navigator will, on occasion, lose their way. All patients, especially during this very difficult adjustment period, appreciate directions and a warm response to any questions they have about where to go. This is a time when individuals feel particularly vulnerable and will value guidance compassionately given.

Loneliness and solitude

It is quite common for individuals to feel lonely in the alien world of the metropolitan city, away from the comfort of their family and friends. Telephone bills can run high as calls home are a vital link to the intimate world of significant others. The nightly call home may be the only connection to family life.

As time passes individuals often begin to develop close relationships with other patients and families at the hospital or at accommodation centres. It is often the case that the closest and most lasting relationships are formed with those who share the early stage of treatment. The personnel at treatment centres also become familiar and bonds develop. Because the treatment protocols are lengthy, there is considerable time for individuals to develop substitute emotional networks at the treatment centres.

Those who take the time to talk and to sit and listen will be appreciated in a world where everyone else seems to be in a rush. Patients and their families need support, encouragement and a sympathetic ear. However, they also need the personal space to deal with their situation. It is often easy to forget that the gift of respecting privacy is just as important as the offer of shared conversation. The escape from loneliness and the desire for solitude can be competing but equal needs.

The special needs of young families

It has been well documented that one of the most emotionally painful experiences associated with oncology is the sheer anguish parents feel when their child is diagnosed with one of these illnesses. Many parents state that it is not possible to put such feelings into words; those who do try use descriptives such as 'an overwhelming and unfathomable grief'. These parents and their families have very special challenges that should be understood by all who care for them.

When a child is diagnosed with one of these conditions, the high level of care demanded of parents necessitates that the needs of the sick child become paramount. This has ramifications for all members of the family, particularly in those families that have to relocate from their home-town for long periods of time. With diagnostic groups such as acute lymphoblastic leukaemia, the protocols stretch over two or more years. For relocated families with young children this can have a profound significance.

For such families the central challenge becomes that of keeping the family unit functioning as normally as possible. This is difficult, to say the very least, when the family becomes split between the treatment centre and their home of origin due to circumstances beyond their control. Siblings, in particular, are affected – this is dealt with in detail in Chapter 5. The lack of choice associated with family separation remains an ongoing core concern. Parents talk of the unresolvable tension of having to be in two places at the one time. Understandably, this is distressing to parents who feel 'trapped by their circumstances' and see no alternatives but to adjust and learn to deal with the situation. The concern is not just about the lack of quality of life for the family but rather about the impact the family disruption will have on the child(ren)'s development.

The research indicates that any efforts made by families to maintain their family life and create special times of closeness for family members will be well rewarded. This is an area where families who have to relocate many miles away from home, particularly when young children are involved, are at a great disadvantage. Some families, who live many hundreds of kilometres from the hospital, wisely and with good results, choose to do the round trips, rather than relocate, in order to keep the family together. Unfortunately, this is not always practically possible.

It is also more difficult for families during the initial intensive stage of therapy (induction remission and consolidation) than during the later maintenance stage, when patients are able to spend longer periods at home. Again, it should be stressed that these are circumstances beyond the control of families and in many ways the only real solution will be the eventual development of community-based back-up medical services which will help to support patients in their own homes.

Conclusion

Uncertainty is the catchword for those who must relocate. Individuals arrive in the city, many having never been there before, uncertain of their exact diagnosis, how long they are going to stay, whether the visit is about diagnosis or involves treatment, where they will be living and how their families will be coping at home. This is a very difficult time, so those going through it need to be mindful of the extraordinary challenge they are dealing with. *To function at all is to be coping very well!*

As can be seen by the detail in this chapter, there are many very real demands placed on individuals and their families at the point of diagnosis and initial treatment. Most people caught in this whirlwind of changes have few choices but to learn to accept the situation and cope. It says a great deal about the strength of the human spirit that people do cope under such odds.

It is far too easy for families coping with this challenge to underestimate their strengths in dealing with the situation. Everyone who passes this way will feel confusion and disorientation and have genuine moments of feeling strained to the limit. Unfortunately, it is quite common to find that others around you, even loved ones, may not understand how difficult it is. It is hoped that, by hearing of the experiences of others, it will help you to feel more 'normal' about your own situation. Take heart in the knowledge that many have come this way before and coped. There is now an increasing recognition of the huge demands placed on families during this time and health care and community organisations are starting to respond with support services to help lessen your load.

Chapter 3

THE EMOTIONAL
ROLLER-COASTER RIDE

There are a wide range of emotional challenges that the patient and
their family will have to face during their journey with this group of
diseases. Although every individual will have their own unique set
of circumstances to deal with, there are a distinct set of emotional
concerns that are common to all.

Uncertainty

One of the key difficulties underpinning the experience is that of the
stress of uncertainty. The uncertainty can start prior to the point of
diagnosis when patients sense that something is wrong but are
unable to have a diagnosis confirmed. During this time, many will
confront their worst fears and will actively seek honest, rather than
comforting, opinion from their doctor. Others, however, will hold
out the hope that the uncertainty will mean that they will not have
their suspicions confirmed.

The uncertainty is not resolved with the labelling of the disease.
Individuals must wait for confirmation of further important variables such as sub-type, the risk (standard or high), and staging. This
is not an area of medicine where definite statements come easily. All
of the important questions such as life expectancy, expected side
effects, and treatment strategies will come couched in uncertain
terms with references to individual variations in disease progression
and response to treatment. It is simply not possible to know in
advance the individual's reaction to treatment, the symptoms they
will display, or the way their body will recover from the drugs and

interventions used. Decisions at each step along the way will depend on the particular circumstances existing at the time. The significance attributed to waiting for test results is an indication of the pressure individuals feel in coping with this pervasive uncertainty.

For those who have to relocate to the metropolitan area for specialist treatment, uncertainty issues escalate. Upon leaving home many do not know where they will stay, how long they will be gone, or when and if there will be return trips home. As described in a previous chapter, uncertainty about issues associated with the hospital and metropolitan environment abound. This sense of uncertainty is reported to be pervasive and permeates all aspects of coping with the treatment experience.

Dealing with this uncertainty is a challenge that is reported to need a flexible approach to life, as the individual has to constantly plan around the demands of treatment. The frustration associated with the impossibility of making reliable plans, even for the immediate future, is one of the significant restrictions of the treatment experience.

Shock

When individuals are given the diagnosis, they and their loved ones will experience a sense of shock that can be both profound and overwhelming. It has been described as similar to 'a bomb going off, when all of a sudden everything around you is affected'. The experience has also been likened to 'one big roller coaster ride that is not going to stop'. Some individuals can pin-point the exact moment the shock really 'hits'. This is usually associated with the discussion of test results with the specialist doctor, but can come with more subtle cues such as a parent of a child patient being asked to go outside the room for discussions with a doctor.

Everyone handles the shock differently. Reactions can vary from immediate anxiety, including sleeplessness and stomach upsets, to denial. Some individuals take time to fully process the implications of the diagnosis and will consciously block thoughts about the situation in an attempt not to be overwhelmed. It is not unusual for individuals to appear in control for a while and then later experience a sense of being overwhelmed. The sense of shock can challenge the individual's sense of normality and it is imperative for them to understand that a profound reaction is to be expected and that the way they feel is 'normal' under the circumstances. It is important for individuals in shock to have their reality affirmed and not be made to cope with the added burden of hearing that the intensity of their feelings is unusual or that the expression of such feeling indicates that they are not coping adequately.

Why me?

One of the really difficult questions often posed is 'Why me?' For many, this will be one of the hardest parts of coming to terms with the fact of the diagnosis. Individuals can feel an irrational sense of responsibility for their disease. The fact that there are very few known causative factors for this set of diseases can make the situation harder, not easier, to deal with. Those affected can feel an intense sense of unfairness and an inappropriate sense of self-blame. To date, with the exception of some conclusive work on radiation and a number of chemicals such as benzene, our understanding of the causation of these diseases is in its infancy. However, recent research indicates that, in comparison to patients with other diseases where the cause is known, the mystery of cancer can leave individuals feeling unrealistically responsible for their diseases. Onlookers, frightened themselves by the unknown, can be all too keen to reinforce this perception because it somehow brings a comforting sense of increased control and predictability thus reducing their own sense of vulnerability.

Coming to acceptance

Most individuals achieve some degree of acceptance of their situation. This acceptance can be seen by such statements as 'you cannot change it so you have to deal with it'. This process cannot be hurried and each individual will need the support and personal space to come to terms with the facts of the disease at their own pace.

Putting life on hold

Many of the treatment protocols extend over years, not weeks or months and so, for most people, this will be a long journey. The sheer length of the time involved can be daunting for many, particularly parents with other young children to worry about. To a large degree, life revolves around the medical drama during this period. Consequently, it is very common for patients and their families to feel as if they have had to 'put life on hold'. Planning for the future is postponed as the demands of surviving the present take precedence.

The emotional roller-coaster ride

Even with a fair degree of acceptance, the emotional journey has been likened to an emotional roller-coaster ride. The metaphor of a roller-coaster is used because the experience has been described as having the ups and downs of feeling good one day but being quite devastated the next. It is not unusual for individuals who seem to be coping one day to spend the next in tears or irritability from the stress of the situation.

There are wide ranges of emotions associated with the ride. There can be great sadness, not only for the patient but also for their loved ones. As explained earlier, even when individuals know that they are being irrational, it is not easy for them to escape the endless soul-searching associated with 'Why me?' or 'Why my child?' For many, this will be coupled with a strong sense of unfairness, particularly when the young are affected.

Especially in the case of the acute diagnostic groups, the treatments can be long, intense and start immediately, leaving the patient and their family feeling overwhelmed and out of control of the situation. Often individuals report a profound sense of lack of choice, as there appear to be few alternatives to treatment and they are carried along by the medical drama. Although most do cope with the demands of treatment, many retain a desire to escape the medical drama, if only momentarily, to have the personal space to sort out their emotions. For many, anxiety, depression and fear can be intense emotions that accompany the treatment experience.

However, it also needs to be acknowledged that individuals bring an array of powerful positive feelings to the illness experience. Hope is a key ingredient in dealing with the diagnosis that motivates individuals to 'give their all' to the treatment experience and creates a sense of optimism about the future. Such optimism is translated into such statements as 'you have got to try and beat it' or 'I want to feel that I have done the best I can'. It is this 'fighting spirit' combined with the perception of the self as survivor that nourishes and sustains individuals during this difficult time.

Remaining positive for others

In spite of the difficulty of the situation, many do feel the need to be strong and positive for others. For this reason, it is not always easy to share the real feelings with close family members. There is the expectation that, where the patient shows the strength to cope, this needs to be supported by a show of positive cheeriness by the carer. This is exacerbated in the hospital situation, which is usually considered to be a place where it is difficult to express emotion. Patients and family members can feel the pressure to 'wear a cheery mask' and hide their real emotions for moments of privacy. This can be very difficult over long periods in the hospital setting and moments of personal space when real feelings can be expressed are usually prized.

The need for emotional release

Maintaining a positive outlook and having encouraging support for others is important to those coping with the demands of treatment. However, most individuals also value the opportunity for emotional release, especially through crying. The chance to express feelings is positive, as it helps the individual to 'off-load a bit' and allows a degree of relief. Although it is common to hear the saying 'men don't cry', the need for tears is not gender specific. This is a time when men and women alike have the need for emotional release.

Patients and close family members appreciate it when others provide the opportunity and encouragement for them to express their real feelings about their situation. Consequently, the often well-meaning urging by others to 'be positive' can lead to feelings of being misunderstood and, to some degree, being patronised. As a parent with a leukaemia child stated clearly, 'there is no bright side when your child has got leukaemia; those who say think positive have never ever had a child have this'. Such invitations to be positive, however, are usually understood as expressions of the discomfort other people feel in the face of such misfortune and the general inability to know how to react or what to say. For many patients, a more helpful response from those trying to offer support is the simple act of acknowledging the difficulty of the journey. The opportunity to share feelings with others can be very therapeutic. Sharing with others that understand not only helps by affirming the individual's reality, but also creates supportive bonds.

Inner strengths

This discussion of the emotional roller-coaster ride does not mean to imply that patients and their families do not manage to find within themselves a positive power to cope. It is impossible to work in this area without being profoundly touched by the remarkable strengths that individuals find in the face of adversity. If individuals are allowed to express their real feelings they will come to understand the positive power in themselves more fully and naturally. Too often, the fear of being trapped in despair prevents both patients and their carers from expressing negative feelings and thoughts. There is a wide-spread belief that if the individual is allowed to express their despair they may lose hope, perhaps to the point of becoming suicidal. Yet, talking about real feelings with someone who under-stands and cares is not a recipe for such disaster, it is an important process for encouraging coping.

Compassionate concern for others

In spite of the emotional challenges the patient and their family are facing, it is quite common to hear expression of compassion for others. There is often a heightened appreciation of the struggle of others, accompanying a deepened understanding of the fragility and preciousness of life. Indeed, many individuals touched by the harshness of this reality find strength, comfort and healing in the process of helping others. The insight and understanding gained from the experience is often made to work for the individual in a very positive way by extending compassion to others in a similar situation.

Conclusion

Each individual will bring a unique life history and set of personal relationships to their treatment experience. The differences will be profound. However, underlying this difference will be a common thread of experience. Others who have not had to face similar difficulties will not readily understand this experience. All too often, people not only have to cope with the strong emotions associated with diagnosis and treatment, but have to do so in a vacuum of understanding where even significant others are unaware of their emotional plight. It is easy in such a situation to whitewash emotions and to provide platitudes as a response. The expectation in writing this chapter is that it will provide a medium through which the complexity of emotions can begin to be understood. This information will affirm the normalcy of the emotional struggle for those who have to cope with these illnesses and will provide insights for those who care. Above all, it is hoped that the information will help all involved to respect and acknowledge as 'normal' the wide range of emotions involved in this journey.

Chapter 4

SUPPORT ISSUES

The importance of support

It is now well understood that the provision of appropriate and timely support can make a very important positive difference to the individual and their family's ability to cope. There is, however, enormous variation in the amount of support available to different individuals and to the same individual at different points in time. Increasingly, community and health care organisations are accepting the responsibility for providing supportive services where there is a demonstrated, but inadequately met, need.

Yet, it is still early days in relation to the development of patient support services. Although there are organisations that provide excellent services, overall the picture is still patchy. It will, to a large degree, still be a matter of serendipity as to whether you are in the geographical location to access appropriate services. It is also hoped that the information from this book will be used to stimulate and inform the need for further support service development.

I know, I care, but what do I say?

One of the most difficult learning experiences that most people face after receiving confirmation of their diagnosis is the realisation that many of their friends and acquaintances do not know how to respond. Coming, as it does, at a time of great vulnerability and increased need to share with others, this realisation can be quite painful. Following is a description of the typical ways people are likely to react to the news of a person being diagnosed with a haematological malignancy.

Unless others have actually had to cope with similar situations in their own lives they will, to a large degree, not have the life experience to understand the significance, or the reality, of a diagnosis of a haematological malignancy. The lack of shared experience is made worse by the fact that many individuals are just unable to face, or deal with, the difficult feelings associated with serious illness. We live in a materialistic consumer society where individuals are bombarded daily with messages that are packaged to provide quick-fix, now-oriented answers to all of life's problems. This is not an environment conducive to listening to the reality of others' struggles. It takes genuine emotional strength to be able to stop and sensitively listen to the concerns of others.

Consequently, it is quite common for individuals to experience genuine disappointment, and at times considerable hurt, when they find significant others in their informal and formal networks of relationships are unable to handle the fact of the illness. The challenge is to not take the inability of others to cope as a personal rebuttal, but to put the reaction in the context of the wider picture of how each and every one of us copes with the reality of illness. Just as some will run away, others will stay and surprise others with their strength.

There are many who can and will want to provide support but are at a loss to know what to say. Such individuals worry about saying the wrong thing for fear that their comments may cause distress. In such a situation, the individual may consider it is better to say nothing rather than to make a mistake. At the other end of the continuum, others can unrealistically take on the responsibility of attempting to make 'everything all right', perhaps by offering encouragement to be positive or by providing advice. These groups share one important thing in common; they do care and want to demonstrate their caring. However, silence, advice giving and the pressure to be positive are all responses that can be problematic to patients. The caring can, however, so easily and appropriately be expressed by the simple act of listening. The courage to stop and hear another's story can be a profound gift of compassion and understanding. Magic wands are not necessary, all that is needed is the humble gift of making the effort to connect and share.

Been there, done that!

There is a third group of people who can provide immeasurable benefit and comfort to others faced with the challenge of *Living with Leukaemia* and these are the individuals who have been through a similar situation. It is very common for patients to seek out such people either in the informal network or through hospital or voluntary group connections. For some, the relationship becomes a deep friendship that grows from the bond of sharing the unique intimacy of a journey that can only be understood by first-hand experience. This friendship provides the comfort zone where questions can be asked, fears revealed, anxieties laid to rest and detailed knowledge gained of the journey that lies ahead. On occasions, such individuals are formally sought and can act as role models and mentors.

However, even these relationships have their limitations, as not all will want to gaze into the crystal ball of other people's experience. There will be those who will fear hearing more than they can emotionally deal with and who will not be nourished by hearing the plight of others. The need for this contact can vary over time, with some individuals delaying contact with others in a similar position until such time as they feel strong enough to cope with the information they hear.

The need for personal space

Lastly, there is the important world of the self. Many individuals, whilst appreciating the comfort of the support provided, will seek the solace of their own personal space. Again, there will be a wide range of individual differences. Many will only require a short time out from the intensity of response that the news of the diagnosis can bring. Others will find that their primary mode of coping will be through the stolen moments of quiet reflection where they can touch base with their inner soul. As with all of these matters, there is no correct or incorrect way of coping, there are just different styles.

The gift of a supportive network

One of the core difficulties in relation to haematological malignancies, that sets it apart from other groups in oncology, is that many of the treatment protocols can be over a very long time, in some cases extending for years. This cannot be a solo journey, it requires the combined efforts of a supportive network.

To survive such a lengthy ordeal all families will require the back-up of family and friends. The support that is available will be tested to a large degree. Without support, any family system will be very fragile and the individuals in it vulnerable to a wide range of coping problems and stress conditions.

This is not a topic where it is appropriate to generalise. There is extensive variation in the support available to families. Some will have extended family networks that can provide practical and emotional support for however long it is needed. Particularly in the rural areas, there can be strong community networks that are capable of generating ongoing interest and strong practical back-up for families. Some schools and employers can and do play exemplary roles of support and demonstrated good will to families during their time of need.

Unfortunately, not all families are so fortunate. Some may have only just moved to a new town prior to the diagnosis and so will not have established reliable contacts. Others may be coping with informal networks fractured by family break-ups or significant bereavements. Many will have their finances so strained by the ongoing medical drama that there will be no comfort zone to buffer the impact. Not all schools or employers respond in understanding ways to the plight of those who have to cope with a haematological malignancy.

Typically, support will be available to most families during the somewhat intense stage of diagnosis and initial treatment. To know that support is there is important and valued, but the individual may need help in handling all the communication associated with keeping supporters in touch with the situation.

As time goes on, such support structures can be difficult to maintain. This is particularly so for families that are forced to relocate for treatment away from the intimate networks of family and home-town friends. Increasingly, health care and community organisations are understanding that this is an important area in which they must play a role.

School and work

I have heard so many inspiring stories of schools going to great length to keep in contact with children who, on a moment's notice, have been relocated to the metropolitan area for specialist treatment. These efforts are always deeply appreciated by both the children and their parents. At a time when the child's whole sense of self and normality is shaken, such contact provides a life-line of support and contact with the familiar world of their pre-hospital experience. Children cherish hand-made artefacts by school friends and often proudly display them in the hospital setting for all to see. Research is starting to show that such contact improves the child's chances of a successful adjustment to, and positive outcome from, their treatment experiences.

Children typically feel a mixture of excitement and anxiety at the thought of returning to school. They look with great enthusiasm to resuming a normal existence and re-connecting with friends. For many, however, their confidence and self-concept can be shattered by an altered body appearance, such as hair loss, and their period of isolation from the world of their peers. Most children return to school with considerable nervousness about the reception they will receive from others. The support of teachers and friends at this point of integration is essential. There are many myths about haematological malignancies, such as that they are contagious or that death is inevitable, that can easily be defused by thoughtful preparation by teachers. Many schools now use puppet shows or storybook reading as an imaginative way to prepare the class for the child's return. All children love to be made welcome and none more so than those who are coping with a haematological malignancy. These children, however, will be sensitive about their difference and will greatly value a return that allows them to take up a 'normal' role as just one of the children in the class. All children have a strong need to fit into the group.

As detailed previously (Chapter 2, *Early Days*), there are wide variations in the responses of employers to the news that a member of their organisation is dealing with a haematological malignancy. Suffice it to say here that employers can play a crucial and much appreciated role in the provision of support to families.

A more detailed discussion of the economic impact of the illness will be dealt with in a later chapter (Chapter 6, *Talking Finance*).

Supportive organisations

Although it is still early days in the development of support services, there are a number of significant initiatives available to those fortunate enough to live in the geographical locations where they are offered.

Accommodation services

Most hospitals now have accommodation units available upon request. Unfortunately, research indicates that most individuals are unaware of these services and many only find out after arriving at the hospital or after requesting information because of the difficulties they are experiencing. It is important to note that there are accommodation services, many free of cost, and that information on these services can be obtained before leaving home. Some of the accommodation villages provide a range of additional services, such as practical assistance, support and educational courses, interest groups and grief counselling.

Educational courses

It is now increasingly understood that the provision of information on the disease, its treatments and strategies to assist coping, can greatly assist patients and their families. Courses are now designed to provide this information in a relaxed and non-threatening environment in which individuals meet with others in a similar situation. Unfortunately, even where such courses exist, patients and their families are often poorly informed about their availability and few health and allied health professionals make regular referrals.

However, those who attend do rate the experience as very satisfying and express appreciation for the information they are given and the opportunity to make contact with others in similar situations. For those developing such courses, the important qualities that participants look for in presenters are warmth, a non-judgmental attitude, a relaxed approach, a preparedness to interact with and listen to others and an ability to share something of their own story with the group. Presenters need to be mindful that sometimes individuals are attending for companionship needs and may not want to be exposed to too much information, or to information that could be potentially distressing. The information individuals seek is not just clinical, but rather, involves understanding the experience of diagnosis, treatment and survivorship. Participants will be interested in the special knowledge and sensitivity they can receive from others who have been through similar situations and are willing to share thoughts about their experience.

Support groups

It is increasingly becoming apparent that one of the most significant forms of assistance for individuals is contact with others going through similar experiences. This contact often happens informally with patients getting to know other patients in the ward at the hospital or parents of sick children linking up with other parents over a cup of coffee in the parents' room. Strong bonds are made at accommodation centres where families can come to know each other whilst carrying out daily chores.

Some centres actively encourage such informal networks by holding morning teas or other social activities. Newsletters and special interest groups can all play a vital role in fostering much-needed supportive relationships. Individuals who have personal experience in the area often express their altruism and compassion by taking the initiative to organise support groups for themselves and others. Also, this is an area where health and allied health professionals are increasingly taking initiative.

Support groups are important not only as an avenue through which individuals can gain access to information, but also because such groups can offer the safe space for exploring feelings, meeting with others and normalising the experience of illness. Dealing with serious illness can be an isolating and lonely experience and individuals can easily feel they are alone with their problems. Meeting with others can provide a more realistic perspective and help the individual to understand that their struggles are 'normal' in the circumstances. The present indications are that participants find support groups most satisfying if the other members have a lot in common. Hence there can be a wide range of support groups such as parent groups, specific diagnostic groups, survivor groups and grief groups. Most people are hesitant and somewhat nervous about joining support groups, but those who do indicate that they are greatly nourished by the experience.

Conclusion

Accessing appropriate support is an important element in *Living with Leukaemia*. Unfortunately, many individuals and their families, for reasons beyond their control, will not have adequate practical and emotional support. This is an area where we have a long way to go. However, the issue is at least now on the agenda and there is an increasing professional and public awareness of the importance of ensuring that assistance is there for those who need it. Such assistance should not only be for practical support, as important as this is, but should go some way to nourishing the spirit. This is an area where stories of courage and strength abound. Hearing and sharing these stories can be both positive and inspirational for all involved.

Chapter 5

DON'T FORGET ME!
THE WELL SIBLING'S LAMENT

The sibling's dilemma

To understand what is happening to families it is important to appreciate that, to a large degree, parents feel powerless in the face of a stressful situation that is beyond their control. This is a time when families have to survive and cope with the myriad of demands thrown at them. Time and resources do not stretch far enough. Everyone in the situation has no choice but to simply cope the best way they can. All family arrangements are *ad hoc* and are usually determined by the demands of the hospital treatment protocol. Consequently, the impact on siblings has largely to do with the situation in which the family members find themselves.

The experiences and concerns of siblings of a child patient are often unwittingly overlooked during the intense family drama of coping with the fact of diagnosis and treatment. For good reasons, it is all too easy for all participants in the drama, both family and health care, to focus predominantly on the plight of the sick individual. Indeed, research is starting to indicate that during the intensity of demands of treatment the whole pattern of family life becomes disrupted. It is just not possible, even with the strongest will in the world, for many families to maintain a balanced response to the needs of all members of the family. Consequently, siblings can miss out on much needed attention.

Special issues for families who relocate

This is particularly so where families have to relocate for specialist treatment. For most families this will be the first time they have ever had to consider the possibility of having to separate. Unlike other significant family decisions, there is no time for slow deliberation of the alternatives. With very short notice parents have to make major decisions such as whether to allow the siblings to remain in the comfort of their familiar home environment or to bring them to the metropolitan centre.

The decision-making will rest on a number of factors, such as the age of the child, an estimation of the emotional impact of separation, the availability of a care-taker parent at home, the disruption to schooling, and the back-up of family and friend networks. Hospitals and accommodation centres are not particularly suitable places for toddlers or young children and so this decision-making can be very difficult for parents with young children. There will be a trade off between the negative effect of the disruption created by withdrawing the sibling from their home environment and the realistic concerns about the effect on the child of the separation from their parent. Parents will be in a vulnerable emotional space when making these decisions as this will be a time when families are in shock and just learning to cope with the turmoil of the treatment experience.

There are a range of choices families make. Some decide to split the family with one parent, or perhaps a grandparent, caring for the siblings at home whilst the other parent relocates to the metropolitan centre. Other families decide to relocate with the whole family for the duration of treatment. Still others travel many hundreds of kilometres in round trips to and from the hospital so that they are able to keep the family together at home. No matter what the decision, this can be a very hard time for both the parents and the siblings.

Parents can experience considerable distress at not being able to continue to be involved in the daily activities of the siblings left behind. There are significant close family times such as bed time, after school and special occasions, that are especially missed. It is common for families to feel a profound disruption to their sense of normal family life. Parents can be very concerned about the long term consequences of separation.

All families are challenged

Even where parents can handle the treatment situation from their own home there is still the ongoing pressure of making arrangements for the care of siblings during the extensive periods when the parent must be at the hospital with the sick child. The support of friends and family is essential. However, even with adequate support parents must face the endless daily arrangements that have to be made at short notice. Such arrangements are made in a continuous state of uncertainty, for the parent can never be sure as to when the sick child will need to go to hospital or how long they will have to stay.

In order to reduce the impact on the siblings of the disruptive experience, parents may take care to present the minding arrangements in a positive light. Young children can be encouraged to feel special about their visit to their grandparents or to look forward to playing with other children at the place they will be looked after. Individuals from within the family or friend network who provide continuous loving care to the children are greatly valued because of the essential stability they provide to the siblings.

It is to be expected that as the parent's time and energy will be deflected to the care of the sick child siblings can feel a sense of abandonment, particularly if relocation is involved. This can lead to anger as well as feelings of bitterness and jealousy. It is not unusual for the well sibling to suffer a sense of guilt for being the healthy one, which can be compounded by having to deal with the jealous feelings created by separation from the parent. Even when the parent returns home, the sheer practical difficulties associated with the care of the sick child can alienate the well siblings. There can be extra demands and limits placed on the sibling, such as restrictions to visitors to the house or the pressure to maintain high levels of cleanliness because of fear of infection. In short, it is easy to see why siblings can be directly and negatively affected at all stages of the medical drama.

Different reactions at different ages

There will be different issues and reactions depending on the age of the child.

Pre-school children are vulnerable because of their young age and dependency on the parent. They are not suited to the hospital environment and accommodation centres. This is particularly so if they are country children used to space in which to play. Because of the intensity of care the parent is required to give to the sick child, it can be very difficult in the hospital setting to focus appropriately on the pre-schooler. Although it is assumed that they are quite limited in their understanding of the medical drama, if the parent provides age-appropriate explanations many do manage to grasp a basic idea of the situation. Indeed, one mother I interviewed reported that her pre-schooler tells friends that the sick sibling has *got sick blood and has to go to the doctors for a long time to make him better.*

Even with the best of arrangements pre-schoolers can feel anger at being left behind. It is not unusual for parents to have to endure an expression of that anger and to see their child shy away from them. On returning home, the parent may feel the need to take steps to re-establish the bond, which may involve acknowledging the anger and, where possible, spending individual time with the child. Fathers often play an increased role in caring for the young children and the bonds that develop can go a long way to balancing the feelings of rejection the siblings may feel. Some parents, however, do manage to actively involve the pre-schooler in the treatment experience.

Although *school age* children are more independent and able to stay at home and remain in school and recreational activities, they also report missing the parents and look forward to the day when treatment will be finished and the family re-united. For school age children the vulnerable times seem to be in the morning before school, after school and at bed time. Both parents and children feel a loss when the parent cannot attend special school or recreational occasions because of hospital commitments. As with all family members, the school age child will have a sense of loss about the disruption to 'normal' family life. In some cases, school age children will choose to take on extra responsibilities in the family because of the absence of the parent. However, others may resent the increased pressure on them to assist with household chores. The school age child will be able to talk about and understand the treatment experience.

Teenage siblings and their parents have their own special set of problems as they try to negotiate the pressures of adolescence with the distraction of a medical drama. The need to self-actualise can conflict with the additional responsibilities in the family. Each individual will handle it differently.

Common feelings

Siblings report that, because of the lengthy treatment protocols, coping with the family disruption for such long periods is very difficult. They can have a range of feelings including sadness about the illness, anger, frustration, disappointment, a sense of being left out, jealousy, negativity, a longing for or sense of missing the parent and a sense of love and protection towards the sick child and their parents. It is quite normal for them to feel both jealousy at the attention the sick sibling receives and guilt at feeling such jealousy when they are the healthy one. However, in spite of the displacement, the siblings will also be feeling concern for the sick family member. Not all children can express this concern directly. Some will express their feelings openly and others will withdraw and deal with the situation by themselves. The presence of a sympathetic, stable adult figure who is available to listen to their feelings and concerns can be of considerable assistance.

Coping strategies

For most families it will be a matter of coping from day to day with the excessive demands placed on them, accompanied by a sense of lack of control over the quality of family life they can maintain. However, the evidence suggests there are strategies that can assist in reducing the problems the siblings will be facing.

Whenever possible, it can help to talk about the sibling's real feelings. Accepting the negative feelings as well as the positive can be a healing process. Once expressed, accepted and understood as normal for the situation, negative feelings can loose some of their power to harm. Most families intuitively try to maintain their home life as normal as possible, in spite of the drama. Any energy placed in retaining a sense of normalcy will have very positive results. In this respect families who have to relocate for treatment have a much more difficult task. Those who have to cope with longer treatment protocols (such as the two or more years of the ALL protocol) will also be at a disadvantage.

It is most important that those families understand that the ability to survive the day-to-day demands placed on them is a very special achievement in itself. This is a difficult journey for any family and it is imperative that expectations about what can be achieved remain realistic. It is hoped that an understanding of what other similar families are going through might help all of those facing this situation to understand that they are not alone in their struggle to meet the needs of their children and that the issues they are facing are shared with others.

Friends and family members can be encouraged to pay attention to the siblings as well as the sick child and to be sensitive to the possibility of focusing too exclusively on the patient.

Here are a list of suggestions from parents as to how to deal with the situation;

- Wherever possible, try to maintain continuity in the care of the child. It can be of great assistance to siblings to be cared for by stable and familiar figures who are able to build significant relationships with them over time. Those families who have regular and sustained support of family and friends will be most fortunate in this regard.
- It can be helpful for parents to be positive about the child-minding arrangements by incorporating a sense of fun. For

example, children can look forward to a visit from their grand-mother or the opportunity to play with friends. Again, the success of this approach will depend on the supportive network available and the creative energy available for planning the care. This is difficult when arrangements have to be constantly made without opportunity for planning.

- Where ever possible try to engage in 'normal' activities. To a large degree, during the intensity of treatment, most family activities will be restricted. However, it is important to take any opportunity to share the special moments associated with the rhythm of family life. It is also important, however, to accept that for the intense period of treatment your sense of what is 'normal' will have to be different to what it was previously. The moments of 'normalcy' are more likely to be a luxury rather than the expected.

- Encourage family and friends to be sensitive to the needs of siblings for attention. A sensitive issue in this regard is the provision of presents for the sick child without consideration for the feelings of siblings. Both family and friends can play an important role in allowing siblings to feel valued and loved. They can also provide the much needed emotional space in which the sibling can talk about the difficulties they are experiencing.

- Where possible, create some individual time for the sibling. It is appreciated that this may not be easy. However any time spent talking or sharing pleasurable activities will be of considerable value.

- Allow the sibling to express their real feelings about the situation and assure them that it is normal to feel such a range of emotions. The opportunity to talk honestly about the situation will help to affirm the sibling's reality and will give them a sense of being listened to.

- Some siblings naturally assume increased responsibility in response to a family crisis. The research indicates that such children can be strengthened by the experience and go on to be very self-reliant adults. It is important to show appreciation for any efforts the child makes. However, not all children are ready or able to shoulder extra responsibilities at an early age.

- Be prepared to be flexible and make compromises. Especially during the intensity of treatment, it will not be possible to maintain the running of the house or the level of social engagement as prior to the diagnosis.

- Above all, accept that you and your child are coping as best you can under the circumstances. This is a difficult time and the problems you are experiencing are very challenging for all those who have to make this journey.

Support services for siblings

Unfortunately, as yet, there are few services that pay attention to the needs of siblings. Hopefully, as our knowledge and understanding of the experience of siblings deepens, more appropriately developed supportive services will become available. This is an area where outside help can be used to complement the resources of the family. The opportunity for siblings to meet and discuss their situation with other children coping with similar demands can be therapeutic. The additional attention of workers who provide creative activities for children and who can provide an ongoing interest in their life would help to provide an emotional safety net for the family. It is still early days in the development of such services, but the hope and expectation is that a creative response to the needs of siblings will be seen in the near future.

Chapter 6

TALKING FINANCE

Financial distress is not an issue that is easily talked about in our society. This may be because the topic is directly related to a wide range of conflicting, and often controversial, beliefs and attitudes about individual versus community responsibility. However, this is an important consideration in relation to families coping with an individual diagnosed with a haematological malignancy, as the treatments are very long and consequently the financial impact can be severe. In our society there is a prevailing ethos that leaves economic viability to the resources of the individual with little understanding of the powerful processes that are outside the individual's control. This chapter is dedicated to all families who have experienced the quite considerable distress of financial hardship as a result of the financial impact associated with the diagnosis and treatment of a haematological malignancy. It is not intended that this be a detailed discussion, but rather that it presents the broad issues to affirm that the economic hardship such families experience is a community not an individual concern.

Additional costs

There will be a wide range of extra costs to the family brought on by the treatment crisis. Travel to and from the hospital, parking, meals, child care arrangements, special foods, pharmaceutical and medical expenses, are but a few of the extra costs for which the family will have to pay. These costs become multiplied for families that have to relocate for specialist treatment as they have also to pay for the running of their home in their absence, long distance telephone calls to home, additional grocery shopping whilst away, and often additional costs in relation to accommodation and travel.

In all states in Australia governments have schemes subsidising travel and accommodation for patients and their carers, but unfortunately these are not well publicised and hence, are under accessed.

Loss of finances

For many families these additional costs will be at a time of loss of income. This happens not only when the 'bread winner' is diagnosed, but also can be a result of the carer having to relinquish their employment in order to be available full time to the patient. This is a particular problem for the self-employed.

In addition to this there is considerable money that is needed 'up front' even if the person is able to claim and be reimbursed at a later date.

Financial buffer

Not every family experiences financial hardship. For some there is a buffer in the form of accommodation and transport assistance, employer or family support, and retirement or insurance benefits. Where the 'bread winner' remains in employment, the carer is able to maintain part-time employment, the family owns their own home or has life savings to call on, then the financial impact can be cushioned.

Long-term problems

It is obvious from this description that those most at risk, for reasons beyond their control, are our young families. Many of these families will not have had the opportunity to build up savings, pay off their home or car, or have mature insurance policies on which to call. The buffer zone of their savings will easily be eroded, particularly if the illness has meant that the family income has been maintained, for some time, at the subsistence level by a pension. The self-employed are also particularly vulnerable.

Financial support

Increasingly community based and health care organisations are beginning to realise and respond to the seriousness of the financial impact of serious illness. This is particularly so with regards to haematological malignancies where the drain on finances happens over years, as the treatments can be prolonged and rehabilitation slow. Such support is vital to families and needs to be extended over the trajectory of the illness, rather than seen as one off interventions.

Conclusion

This short chapter has been included to highlight the financial needs of families. It is hoped that those who are so affected will take heart from hearing that others are in a similar situation and will find the confidence to seek help when needed. It is also hoped that this chapter will be read by the broad range of professional and lay persons who are involved in responding to the financial plight of families so that they can fully appreciate that this situation is out of the individual's control.

Chapter 7

POST-TRAUMATIC STRESS

As can be seen by the challenges outlined in previous chapters, there are many significant stresses associated with *Living with Leukaemia*. It is easy to understand that there is a danger that individuals, for reasons beyond their control, can have an overload of stress. In recent years there has been some innovative work in oncology looking at the symptoms of a condition known as Post-traumatic Stress Disorder (PTSD), which can occur when individuals are exposed to severe acute or prolonged stress. It has been my experience that both patients and their carers can suffer from symptoms of PTSD whilst unaware of what is happening to them. All too often they carry a sense of confusion and disturbance about their emotional state. Just the simple act of finding out about PTSD and its relevance to their situation can go a long way to making people feel comfortable about what they are experiencing. This chapter is dedicated to all those who have had to stretch too far, are feeling worried about their emotional state and who need to know that what they are experiencing has a name, is to be expected and is 'normal' in the circumstances.

The symptoms

PTSD has previously been associated with the impact of obvious traumatic stressors such as natural disasters or war. It is only in very recent years that it has been understood in relation to the experience of cancer. This condition is understood to exist where symptoms of acute stress last for longer than a month after the stressful event. There are four categories of stress symptoms usually considered and these include repeatedly reliving the traumatic event, avoidance of cues reminding the individual of the event, a numbing of general responsiveness and a state of increased arousal. The person can feel dissociated from reality.

In lay terms that can mean that the individual may have times when they actually feel that they are going through a stressful experience that they had in the past all over again. Some people may, for example, be driving along in the car and quite unexpectedly feel that they are back in the hospital undergoing an aspect of treatment they found quite difficult. Or a carer may relive an emotional scene they had experienced whilst looking after a loved one. The 'flashbacks' or reliving of the event, will seem quite real to the individual and may persist over time.

Understandably, such individuals may find themselves avoiding any reminders of unpleasant experiences. They will take the long way around the city rather than go past the hospital or may turn off the radio if a program on cancer comes on. One of the very real difficulties of doing research in this area is that those who are experiencing the symptoms quite genuinely do not want to talk about it. The silence makes it difficult for others to know what is going on and to help.

Individuals so affected often present as emotionally 'flat' and have a lack of interest and numbness in relation to their life and their relationships to others. It is as if they are distracted and all of their emotional energy is consumed processing the stress they have been through. It is easy for those around them to misread such difficulties as being aloof, distant, or uninterested, when in fact the individual is preoccupied with simply coping with everyday life.

There can also be a heightened sense of arousal. Such individuals may jump with fright when interrupted or have an agitated or nervous energy. Physiologically speaking, the individual may have physical symptoms such as increased blood pressure. In such a state people can easily become aggressive and annoyed by incidents they may previously have ignored.

Lastly, there may be evidence of what is called a dissociative state. This is a distressing space where the individual does not quite feel connected with life but is somehow a spectator. Previous simple pleasures will be difficult to experience and the person may find it difficult to connect with others in close and sharing relationships. It is as if they are on the outside of life looking in.

With the combination of these symptoms, which can be experienced in varying degrees, a person can have a sense of feeling strange and as if something is quite wrong, without necessarily know what it is. Troubled by such symptoms, people can retreat into their own world and fail to communicate effectively with others. It is important for them to know that their symptoms are understandable and that it is okay to share what they are experiencing with others.

Vulnerability

Although this area is still new, there are already indications that considerably more cancer patients experience symptoms related to PTSD, as compared with the general population. As yet, definite conclusions, cannot be drawn as to the specific individuals who will be most vulnerable, but there are a number of factors implicated at present.

PTSD is a condition where acute stress is caused by a frightening event that happens outside the control of the individual and is associated with the threat of physical injury or death of the self or a loved one. Consequently, in oncology, PTSD symptoms can be linked to the experience of severe symptoms, difficult treatments, or strong side effects from treatment. A particularly vulnerable time for individuals is during the recurrence of the disease, known as relapse, following treatment. Those who have had prolonged hospitalisation, particularly if it involved time spent in intensive care, are especially at risk.

Emotional support and material comfort can be a buffer reducing the likelihood and intensity of such symptoms. Consequently, patients who lack sufficient social and family support or who do not have material and financial security are also at increased risk. The possibility of suffering PTSD symptoms increases where the individual experiences a succession of traumatic events, such as significant loss and grief, retrenchment, or family separation. In fact, those who perceive their lives to be very difficult and unsatisfying will be more at risk than those who have had a predominantly comfortable life experience. A previous history of PTSD in the family will also increase the individual's chances of having these symptoms. Other risk factors include younger age during diagnosis and treatment and a more anxious personality.

Work in this area is still in its infancy and it is difficult to draw firm conclusions. This is partly attributable to the fact that it is a highly unreported area as those who have the symptoms do not want to talk about their experiences. However, there is an increasing recognition that many are affected and that it is imperative to develop supportive strategies to assist those individuals to understand their emotional situation. Often patients or their care-givers will not exhibit symptoms until the treatment ordeal is over. Due to the nature of the symptoms, the sufferers of PTSD are highly unlikely to seek counselling support because of their need to avoid contexts associated with the stress. For the patients, such symptoms can lead to poor recovery and a tendency to avoid further medical treatments. Consequently, there are many reasons why it is important to begin to understand this phenomenon and to communicate the message that others will understand if an individual is struggling with these symptoms.

A number of supportive interventions have been developed to respond to the needs of individuals experiencing post-traumatic stress. These interventions range from one to one counselling sessions to group work where individuals are provided with the opportunity to meet and talk with others sharing the same problem. Individual counselling can be an important first point of contact, particularly for the individual reticent about sharing their problem. Such individualised contact can allow the person to name and understand their condition. However, research is starting to indicate that support groups, that allow individuals the non-judgmental space to talk about their problems and which focus on finding solutions with others in a similar situation, are highly effective strategies of intervention.

Conclusion

Understanding patients and their families' response to the stress of treatment through an understanding of PTSD symptoms provides promising new insights for supportive care in cancer. Although it is only early days and a great deal of work still needs to be completed to fully understand issues of prevalence and vulnerability, a start has been made. It is important for individuals affected to hear the normalising message that such a reaction to trauma is an expected and potentially remedial aspect of their illness or caring experience.

Chapter 8

GRIEF MATTERS

From the very moment that patients start to have to deal with the troubling symptoms associated with the diagnosis of a haematological malignancy, they and their families begin to experience emotions of loss and grief. Some will eventually have to face the profound grief of losing a loved one. Unfortunately, we live in a society that does not know how to handle these feelings. Most people are under-confident and nervous about responding to any expression of grief. Myths and misconceptions relating to the process of grief abound. Because grief involves very intense emotions, often the normal expression of the pain of loss is 'pathologised', that is, made to appear somehow abnormal. Those who are coming to terms with loss have enough to deal with without having to handle all of the inappropriate, and at times hurtful, comments of others who are struggling to understand what they are going through. This chapter is written to convey basic information about the process of grief so that individuals who are grieving, and those who care for them, have a solid foundation of understanding on which to build their strategies for coping.

The discussion focuses on those who have suffered a significant bereavement but the insights apply to the varying forms of grief associated with confronting and dealing with serious illness. There are aspects of loss that occur from the moment of diagnosis along the continuum of treatment. Grief is not necessarily about bereavement but can be associated with a wide range of life changes such as loss of employment, or altered body image.

The need to talk

Many individuals will have a strong need to talk about their feelings of grief and their experience of coming to terms with their loss. This is often repetitive talk where the person needs to go over the same topic time and time again. Consequently, it is quite usual for families and friends to demonstrate a limited capacity to sustain such intensity and repetitiveness. Some individuals live alone and do not have intimate relationships to confide in. Consequently, there is a great need for support groups and counsellors to provide the space in which those coping with loss can have the opportunity to work through their most pressing issues. Those caring for loved ones in grief need to be reassured that the endless repetition is to be expected and is not an issue of concern. Those who take the time to stop and listen offer an important and special gift.

Not everyone wants to or is able to talk

It must be noted, however, that not all individuals cope by talking and some require a great deal of personal space in which to process their feelings.

Although a generalisation, there is some truth in the fact, that in our culture, men can find it difficult to express feelings. The strong message that 'boys don't cry' is too often internalised and lack of practice in expressing feelings can leave many men with few skills to deal with grief. It is all too easy for the individual to present as though everything is fine, whilst on the inside burdened with a heavy load of unexpressed grief. Men are less likely to go to counselling or support groups and have a much higher suicide rate than women. A man I once interviewed summed up the situation when he stated, 'we say "I am fine" whilst inside we are hurting like hell but do not admit it. We are not really good at saying I really could do with some help and yet we would be much better off if we did'. Men's issues are starting to be placed on the agenda, and it is hoped that this situation will begin to change in the future. In the meantime, it is important to be cognisant of the fact that we all have different styles of dealing with grief and some may need more understanding and encouragement in their efforts to talk about what they are going through than others.

The family context

Consideration also needs to be given to the fact that those caring for the grieving are often grieving themselves. Research indicates that the stress of dealing with the impact of a significant bereavement can have a ripple effect, potentially disturbing all members of a family and their informal networks. All family relationships can be affected as grief can stir up unresolved conflicts. It can be a time of fragility and tension for all involved. The paradox is that at the very time that the family is most needed, it can also be at its most vulnerable. Slowly the health care system is beginning to have a deeper appreciation of the necessity of providing adequate supports, both formal and informal, to bolster the strength already available in family and community networks.

The unrealistic expectation to 'Get over grief quickly'

Much of the early work published on the stages of grief was important in that it initiated a public interest in bereavement and created an increased awareness of the complexity of the emotions involved. However, the notion of a set of definite stages of grieving brought with it an expectation that bereavement is a finite process that can be resolved and completed. In our 'quick-fix' society, this notion can easily be translated into the expectation that individuals can and should 'get over' their grief quickly. The popular expectation is that, if individuals do not quickly resolve their grief, something is wrong.

Even individuals who are coping with profound loss, such as the death of a loved one, are prematurely told that they 'should be over that now' or should be able to 'get on with life'. It is not unusual for such statement to be made within the short time-frame of six to twelve months, a period of time when, for many, the full reality of the grief is just starting to be realised. Although well meaning, such expectations can be confusing, undermining and hurtful for those dealing with the intensity of emotions associated with grief. The end result is that individuals learn not to talk about their concerns, yet this does not act to diminish the grief.

There is a great deal of work associated with the process of grieving. Indeed, some individuals are challenged to completely reconstruct the meaning in their lives. This takes time and individuals so affected require support and understanding from others.

The intensity of the experience

Individuals may experience acute physical and emotional reactions to loss. The physical symptoms can include nausea, sleeplessness, weight loss and somatic pain. There are a wide range of emotional reactions other than sadness, including anger, guilt, regret, resentment, confusion, denial, unfairness, despair, and a heightened sense of one's own mortality. Because most people in our society are not comfortable talking about grief, those who do understand the depth of the emotions are rarely heard. Hence there can be fairly superficial attitudes and beliefs about what is involved. Very few are prepared for the depth of emotional pain that significant grief can create. Because the feelings are not talked about or validated, affected individuals may feel that they are 'going mad' or not coping as well as they should be under the circumstances. As one participant in a grief program commented, 'this is something you do not get a practice run at, it is the one thing in life you do not know what to expect'.

Without an understanding of the complexity of emotions associated with the grieving process, individuals can feel overwhelmed and trapped in despair. Unless individuals know that they will eventually build a new life and the intense feelings of despair will subside, they can truly believe that they 'will never feel any better'. Grief is not a rational process, it involves the emotions and hence requires insights and knowledge about what is happening at the psychological level. Understandably, research indicates that if individuals have information on the experience of grief it can help them to cope.

You will feel better

It is most important to convey to grieving individuals the message that they will not feel as they presently do forever. Although the emotions are intense, they will eventually feel differently. It is often the fear of being trapped in despair, not the despair itself, which can do the most harm. People will particularly need to hear this message during the early months of bereavement.

The space to talk about real feelings

As discussed previously, grief is not just about sadness, it touches on a wide range of human emotions. It is essential for people dealing with grief to be able to talk about their emotions in a non-judgmental atmosphere where they can express and have acknowledged their real feelings about the loss. In some cases, friends and family are not able to provide this space as they are too intimately and emotionally involved. Others who have been through a similar experience can be of great assistance in providing the understanding needed. Certainly, this is an area where there is an important role for grief groups and counsellors. It is important for individuals to talk freely with someone who can understand the complex emotions they are feeling. Often just the naming of the emotion and discussing how it is affecting the individual's life can free the person from a sense of being trapped and allow them to 'move on'. Sympathetic listeners are greatly valued by individuals coping with grief. Such people are not required to have 'the answers to problems' but only the patience to hear another's story and respond with compassion. Warmth, caring and a little laughter can go a long way to helping an individual come to terms with their sense of loss.

Yes, you are normal!

The grief experience can be difficult, not only because of the intense feelings it evokes, but because it can leave the individual feeling that they are somehow abnormal, or not coping. Dealing with the intensity of grief is exacerbated in our society, as grief is still taboo and there is neither understanding nor validation of the process. Even those with friends and relatives to turn to may find them unwilling to talk. The loneliness and isolation can only add to the problems already experienced.

Talking honestly to others going through a similar situation can be very affirming as it will help the individual understand the commonalities in the experience. The most therapeutic aspect of any nourishing relationship is the sense of being understood and accepted for who you are and whatever space you are in. Those coping with grief are in great need of such understanding and acceptance.

Planning ahead

We have moved a long way from seeing the grief associated with a profound loss as a series of stages whereby the individual somehow resolves the grief and resumes their previous normal life. It is now understood that life will be invariably altered and the memory of the deceased will always occupy a space in the new life of the bereaved. The challenge is to build an existence that comes to terms with what happened but allows for a new and different future. In the early stages of bereavement, most individuals will fear that they may never feel any better and may not be able to envisage a new future for themselves. This state of being has been described as 'not being able to see the light at the end of the tunnel'. Those experiencing these feelings need to be reassured that the intensity does pass. A time will come when there will be the motivation and energy to begin planning for the future. Such plans may initially be as minor as rearranging a room in the house or as major as starting a new job or educational course. It is important to value each achievement as a small step forward in the new journey. However, it is often easier to see the progression in retrospect.

Compassion and the desire to help others

It is easy in any discussion of grief to focus on the difficult emotions and make the assumption that there is nothing positive associated with the experience. However, I have found both in my research and counselling experience that one of the dominant themes expressed by those who have suffered the pain of loss is their heightened compassion and desire to help others. Indeed, many find it very therapeutic to help themselves by helping others. There are ample examples of individuals who have used the insights and understanding they have gained from their own difficult experiences to advance the plight of others. It is not uncommon to hear individuals talk of achievements they have made that they would never have contemplated doing if they had not been challenged by the pain of loss.

Conclusion

All of us are touched in some way by loss and grief. For some, the loss can be profound and untimely, such as the death of a partner or a child. Dealing with such bereavement can greatly challenge the individual's emotional and intellectual resources, but can also surprise the individual with their strengths and capabilities. As a society, we need to deepen our collective understanding of the experience of grief and learn to respond sensitively, with compassion and respect. It is hoped that the information in this chapter will make some contribution in this regard.

Chapter 9

LIFTING THE TABOO –
A DISCUSSION ON SEXUALITY

Introducing a discussion on the topic of sexuality is considered diffi-cult, not only for patients and their families but also for health profes-sionals. Consequently, this is an area of functioning that usually receives little attention either in the literature or in practice. However, sexuality is a significant aspect of life and it is now known that it can be especially vulnerable to disruption during serious illness.

The shortness of this chapter reflects the paucity of information that is available on this topic. It would be very satisfying to be able to report lots of insightful information that could assist people to deal with these issues. Instead, the only achievable aim of this chapter can be to begin to *lift the taboo* by putting sexuality on the agenda as an area that needs exploring. It can be definitely stated, however, that it has become increasingly obvious through my research and counselling experience that concerns regarding sexual-ity are of paramount importance to patients and their significant others. However, the concerns will only begin to be addressed if individuals find the courage to begin to talk about their problems and if health and allied health professionals discover the profes-sional confidence to deal with the issues. The following chapter is written in the hope of fostering and stimulating the much-needed dialogue in this area.

Physical changes

To date, most of the research in relation to sexuality and haemato-logical malignancies has focused on reporting the physical changes that an individual can undergo because of the disease and its treatments. It is well documented that both of the modalities used to treat haematological malignancies, chemotherapy and radiation, can cause damage to the individual's sexual and reproductive capacity. There will be great individual variation depending on such variables as the dose and type of drugs used and the location and total dose of radiation.

The physical changes can lead to sexual difficulties and dysfunction. The dominant male concerns are impotence/erectile difficulties, infertility, low sexual desire and altered body image. The dominant female concerns include worries about sterility, femininity, and loss of menstruation. The reports in the research are mixed with some studies claiming no dysfunction whilst others cite decreased libido and sexual dysfunction in as many as half the survivors two or three years off treatment. However, there is evidence to indicate that a substantial proportion of patients with haematological malignancies will experience some form of sexual difficulty associated with the disease and its treatment. Either during or immediately after many of the intensive treatments, such as high dose chemotherapy or bone marrow transplants, there can be a decrease in both interest in, and satisfaction with, sexual activity. This phase can be transitory and the research indicates that, with time, most individuals will return to a level of interest and satisfaction similar to what they were experiencing pre-treatment.

Loss of ovarian function and spermatogenesis can result from treatment. Consequently, concerns about infertility can be paramount for many at child-bearing age and can be a source of considerable grief. Some studies indicate that infertility is reported as the single most upsetting consequence of treatment. Individuals can face a wide range of challenges, from having to deal with the inability to have children to deciding whether to use IVF procedures. It is becoming increasingly common for patients to have their sperm or eggs collected prior to treatment for use in such reproductive technologies. There are survivors who go on to have children after treatment.

Research indicates that it is common for patients to be unaware of the physical status of their reproductive system after treatment.

Many survivors are not even aware of whether or not they are infertile from the treatment. It is important for those so affected to know that appropriate medical attention can go a long way to ameliorating distressing side effects. This follow-up is unlikely to be routinely offered. Thus, this is definitely an area where individuals need to be assertive in gathering information from health professionals, because advice and factual information will not be freely offered.

Sexual identity

Although such information on the physiological changes is important, it fails to build an understanding of the significant emotional and relationship issues individuals face. An individual's sexuality is intimately related to the core of their identity. For many, it can be a significant medium through which affection, closeness and commitment can be expressed.

Perhaps one of the most difficult problems the individual must face is the change to their body image. Not only does the disease create changes, many of the treatments can also cause alterations to the body, such as hair loss and weight fluctuations. Such alterations can affect an individual's self-confidence and challenge their sense of sexual identity. It is reported that many individuals react to the problem by changing their social habits and restricting their social activities.

These problems, however, are not insurmountable and individuals do develop strategies for adjusting. Research on sexuality indicates that the greatest help in coping with the consequences of treatment come from family, friends and supportive partners. For many, their own confidence and inner strength are the important contributing factors in helping them cope. This is an area, however, where talking to someone outside the intimate circle who understands the issues can be of assistance. The topic of sexuality should be included in support group discussions so that individuals are able to share their concerns in a non-judgmental setting with others and be provided with the opportunity to hear how others are dealing with the issue. Just the knowledge that problems in this area are common and expected can help some individuals in their attempt to deal with their concerns about sexuality. It is important to communicate the message that the notion of what is 'normal' needs to be redefined in the context of serious illness. It is also important to stress that the expression of an individual's sexuality can be through intimacy and affectionate touch and does not have to be restricted to the physical act of sexual intercourse. Research indicates that for individuals who are post-treatment, even where there are problems with physical sexual functioning, the ability to give and receive affection remains high.

Insufficient professional support

It is now known that there should be professional interventions targeted quite specifically at those in need. This should not just involve information giving but should include the provision of supportive, counselling relationships that allow individuals to talk through issues at their own pace. There is a particular need for post-treatment counselling to educate and reassure patients and their partners. The services of gynaecologists and endocrinologists are presently under-resourced and should be seen as a routine aspect of follow-up. To date, unfortunately, such professional services are not readily available and so the individuals affected will need to be assertive about their needs.

Seeking help

Too many individuals continue to suffer in silence with concerns that can be remedied through the provision of appropriate medication, adequate information, and sensitive counselling. It is important for those affected to actively seek out information and find counsellors with whom they can discuss issues of concern.

It is hoped that health and allied health professionals reading this book will become cognisant of the need for services in this area and will demonstrate leadership in establishing much needed supportive services.

Conclusion

This chapter has provided a brief overview of the work in the area of sexuality. The information available to date indicates that patients and their partners can experience difficulties in their sexual relationships. Perhaps of even greater importance is the research that indicates that, even though there may be problems with physical sexual functioning, the ability to give and receive affection remains high. Achieving satisfying sexual relationships in spite of such obstacles is possible, for sexuality does not only relate to an individual's physical appearance, but, more importantly, involves their total being including their warmth, caring, maturity, personality, talents and sense of humour.

Chapter 10

POWERING ON – SURVIVOR ISSUES

The recent advances in the care and treatment of haematological malignancies means that greater numbers of patients are now achieving cure, or at least substantial lengths of time in remission. It is still early days, however, in terms of documenting the experience of survivorship and there are considerable gaps in our knowledge. Myths and hasty speculations abound and even the information that has been gathered is still somewhat contradictory. However, this chapter will begin to outline what we know and provide insights from the experience of those who are already travelling the road of survivorship.

The myth of the typical survivor

A great deal has been talked and written about the characteristics of survivors. There is a popular conception that survivors are 'fighters' who because of their 'positive approach' are able to 'beat the odds' and live much longer than others. It would be satisfying to state that there is conclusive proof of such a view, but unfortunately, to date, the research completed on the topic is quite contradictory. Some work indicates that hopefulness has a survival value, whilst other studies show that fighting spirit as a coping style does not extend survival. The danger in the notion is that it can set quite unrealistic expectations for individuals and can be responsible for 'blaming the victim' when survivorship is not achieved. There are many other factors other than the patient's outlook that determine survival, and the research indicates that perhaps one of the most important is the nature and progress of the underlying malignancy. It is thus dangerous to be too dogmatic about the survival myth. Too high an expectation that the patient be ever positive may only add to the burden they are carrying and may limit the degree they can share their real feelings about what they are going through.

The myth of survivorship

Until very recently, another idea that was dominant in regards to those who had completed treatment was that once the medical drama was over then all was well and life could return to normal, exactly as it was before.

There is some truth to this idea as many individuals post-treatment do return to their families and re-establish their work, educational or leisure activities. Some studies show that a majority of survivors are emotionally well adjusted and share an optimistic outlook on life. The research that follows individuals many years after treatment is beginning to reveal a picture of increasing numbers of survivors leading meaningful lives with a renewed appreciation of being alive. There is evidence of substantial numbers returning to the work force, becoming parents, undertaking educational programs, and finding satisfying new directions in life.

Many who were well supported during their illness can come to feel closer to their family and friends. It is not unusual for such individuals to experience a heightened sense of gratitude and a stronger appreciation of the importance of loved ones. It has been shown that many survivors of serious illness show a greater maturity, more patience and tolerance, and no longer take health for granted. It is also very common for those who have suffered through confrontation with serious illness to find in their hearts an increased compassion and understanding of the plight of others. Much of the energy and initiative for the establishment of the much needed support and voluntary groups, that so ably assist others, comes from those who are rebuilding their lives post-treatment.

However, this is only part of the picture. As discussed in the previous chapter on post-traumatic stress some individuals are severely emotionally affected by the trauma of diagnosis and treatment and may need informal and professional support to assist their recovery. Emotional health is the slowest to recover as many patients and their families do not begin to deal with their feelings until the medical drama is over and the patient's physical health begins to build. The first year of recovery can be critical, as individuals are impatient to regain their full strength and are eager to start to deal with the many emotional issues that have been postponed during the crisis of treatment. For many, energy levels are slow to return, fatigue persists and this can make individuals prone to depression. Fatigue is a particular problem where patients are not warned about how long it can take to regain strength or have unrealistic expectations of the recovery period.

Not everyone sees himself or herself as 'back to normal'. For many returning to work can be a distressing experience of discrimination, accompanied by the struggle to keep up an appearance of coping in an environment where there is little understanding or sympathy. Others do not find the physical strength to return to work and have to develop a totally new life style. There can be a difficult adjustment period as the individual grieves their lost potential and has to let go of previously satisfying directions in life. Some may feel a sense of loss of identity as they struggle to understand how they will again take their place in the world.

For reasons beyond their control, not all families are resilient to the stresses associated with serious illness. As discussed previously, siblings are particularly vulnerable to long term adjustment problems. Also, the evidence indicates that, sadly for some, divorce and the fracturing of family life can be a direct result of the severe emotional strain of diagnosis and treatment. Intimate relationships can be challenged by increased difficulties in interpersonal relationships and problems dealing with an altered sense of sexuality. Changed body image, decreased interest in sexual activity, and problems with infertility are all factors which can contribute to partnership breakdowns. This can be compounded by a reluctance to name problems and an inability to talk honestly about concerns. Unfortunately, there is scant literature around that prepares individuals or their partners for the problems they may face.

Most importantly, however, once confronted with the diagnosis of a serious illness the affected individual will always have an altered sense of reality. Thus, survivors may experience a tenuous sense of longevity, which can produce anxiety, uncertainty and depressive ideas. The fear of recurrence can be a major issue, often in the background, but always there. We do not live in a society that is comfortable talking about issues surrounding death or dying and so, all too often, these issues have to be dealt with in a vacuum of silence.

Strategies for coping

This is not a 'how to' book that can provide stock answers to problems such as survivorship. Unfortunately, to date we are only just beginning to ask the right questions to find out what the challenges are. However, the discussion can provide insights from others who have 'been there done that' and hence have wisdom to report. Ultimately, however, each person's response to the situation will depend on a myriad of factors such as the resources they have available, the level of support they receive from others, and the access they have to supportive services.

It is now known that information is crucially important to assist individuals in rebuilding their lives. Realistic expectations assist rehabilitation and coping, as those with overly optimistic expectations can experience disappointment, disillusionment and loss of morale. A good example of this is in the area of fatigue. Those who are recovering from a bone marrow transplant and realise that it may take well over a year before energies return are more likely to pace themselves and feel less disheartened about their restricted activities than those who believe recovery will only take weeks or months. Similarly in the area of sexual dysfunction, individuals may endure in silence a wide range of conditions that are remediable by medical intervention. It is still early days in terms of information provision to survivors so this is an area where individuals will need to be assertive and seek out the information they need.

Perhaps the single most important strategy survivors indicate is important in making a successful adjustment post-treatment is that of accepting an altered sense of normalcy. The challenge is not to return to your pre-diagnosis self, but rather to accept and build on your new reality. Some individuals build on their deepened appreciation of life and heightened awareness of the value of their close relationships by embarking on a less hectic life style that allows for quiet reflection and the possibility of savouring the moment. Others find educational, occupational or leisure pursuits to invest their time and energy in that are more tailored to their present physical and emotional strengths and abilities. The key ingredients to successfully embarking on the new journey, however, seem to be to accept limitations, learn to pace yourself, reconnect with previous or try to find new satisfying activities, find the time and space for personal reflection, and foster meaningful connections with others who understand your journey.

In no way is this seen as an easy task. Any changes in life, particularly those forced upon the individual, involve a degree of grief. Sadness, regrets, depression, a sense of loss are as normal in such a journey as the satisfaction involved in rebuilding a new life. It is most important to be able to share the wide range of emotions with someone who will understand. Unfortunately, because of the myths of survivorship and the generalised reluctance to deal with difficult emotions that is pervasive in our society, the task of finding a sympathetic listener may be more difficult than it first seems. Survivor groups, counselling support, and informal links with others going through the same situation can be of inestimable value for those dealing with survivor issues. Many are at first reluctant to make such connections, for fear of the unknown and because of a need to see themselves as always in control and not needing help. It must be remembered that it is a sign of real strength to seek a connection with others during difficult times. All too often individuals struggle with their adjustment issues with a sense of aloneness and an unexpressed despair that they are somehow inadequate or abnormal. It is all too easy to feel isolated and not coping. Relationships with others who understand or are sharing the same journey will provide the appropriate reference point where the individual can let go of the myth of 'normalcy' and hear from others about the wide range of quite difficult challenges involved in survivorship.

This is not to argue that individuals post-treatment do not cherish the opportunity to take a break from the intense drama of their illness and the exclusive focus on their medical condition. Any activity that allows the individual to live fully in the here and now, and to re-enter life through satisfying pursuits and positive connections with others, is of great significance and value. The opportunity to re-engage meaningfully with life is as important as the chance to talk about feelings associated with the illness. Many will, quite simply, be eager to close the door on their illness experience. The defence mechanism of denial, once seen as a neurotic reaction to stress, is increasingly understood as a helpful and healthy way of dealing with situations that demand on-going and long-term adjustments to distressing life situations. Indeed, the research is beginning to show that those who do well have the ability to reflect on both the positive and negative aspects of life. At one and the same time, such individuals are able to explore in great depth their despair and unhappiness, whilst finding positive strategies to re-enter life and take time out from their situation.

Conclusion

In recent times there has been a significant deepening of our understanding of the issues in relation to survivorship. No longer is it possible to subscribe to the myth that everything returns to normal after treatment and that individuals no longer need sensitive care and support. It is now understood that, indeed, it is at this very point that emotional difficulties that have been cast aside during the intensity of the treatment experience can surface and have to be dealt with. As well, individuals have to face the challenge of rebuilding their lives. Good information, the support of family and friends, professional help, and links with others going through similar situations are all vital aspects of fostering the individual's ability to cope at this stage. It is essential to provide those undertaking this journey the opportunity to express their real feelings, have their difficulties validated, and in so doing, have their sense of 'normalcy' appropriately re-defined.

In sharing their journey with others in the same situation they will be in good company. For anyone entering this path of life is likely to bring a heightened appreciation of what is of value in life and a deep appreciation of the struggle of others.

Chapter 11

THE CONTINUUM OF CARE

In the treatment of all illness there is a continuum of care that embraces both cure and palliation. Most people are aware of the notion of cure. Indeed, most of the anxious questions that are asked with regard to haematological malignancies relate to whether the disease is curable, the success rates of treatment and how long the individual will be expected to live. Although there may be a problem with the interpretation of the word 'cure' (with the medical profession working on the assumption it means being disease free for five years and the lay public thinking it means permanent elimination of the disease), there is still a shared idea that it means to rid the body of the disease.

The same cannot be said for the notion of palliation. Few people have a clear idea of palliative care. This is in spite of its great significance to all individuals diagnosed with a haematological malignancy and their families. The purpose of this chapter, then, is to introduce the reader to the basic concepts of palliative care so that they are sufficiently informed to be able to ask the right questions to obtain the services they need. This is important information that could make a difference to both the individual affected by the disease and their loved ones, so I entreat you to read on.

What is palliative care?

Palliative care starts at the point of diagnosis and refers to all of those interventions that are designed to support and comfort the individual and their family. The palliative focus is not exclusively on the physical body, but rather embraces a broad (the term used is 'holistic') range of issues with regards to quality of life for both the patient and their

67

loved ones. The care offered will involve symptom management and pain relief, as well as emotional and social (the term used is 'psycho-social') support for both the patient and the family.

At the beginning of treatment such care can involve the reduction of distressing symptoms, for example through drugs to reduce nausea; the management of pain associated with medical proce-dures, for example general anaesthetics for lumbar punctures; and the provision of supportive services, for example travel, accommo-dation or counselling services. Such services are offered within the curative system and aim to ensure that the patient and carer are provided optimum support whilst they deal with the challenges of the treatment regimen.

Towards the end of life such care embraces not only the quality of living but also the quality of the dying experience. The palliative care philosophy is respectful of the individual's right to die with dignity and to choose where and with whom this might be. Highly skilled and sensitive hospice teams are available to provide twenty-four hour, seven day a week support either within an in-patient facility or in the patient's home. The focus of hospice care includes not only the patient but also the family, and extends for a year into the bereavement period.

A well kept secret!

Palliative care and hospice services are now well established around the world and research shows a high degree of satisfaction with the care they provide. Unfortunately, however, the research also indi-cates that as yet very few people with haematological malignancies are referred appropriately, if at all, to such services. Indeed, the significant contribution that such services can provide to patients with a haematological malignancy and their families is one of haematology's best kept secrets!

It is far more likely for a patient from one of these diagnostic groups to end life in an intensive care unit rather than in the comfort of their own home surrounded by their loved ones. With appropriate knowledge and careful planning this need not be so.

But I could never cope at home

One of the chief reasons people give for not looking for alternatives to the hospital end-of-life care is that they strongly believe that they could never cope with providing the care at home. Although most patients do not want to be in hospital they at least feel they are safe places where their medical needs can be met. Similarly, although many carers would by choice want their loved one at home, they feel frightened and often overwhelmed by the thought of having to provide the care.

Hospice care is based on the notion of providing seven-day a week and twenty-four hour care for patients and their families. Nursing or medical advice is only a telephone call away and community nurses can attend the home as often as needed. Trained volunteers are the mainstay of the hospice movement and are invaluable in the support they can provide, which ranges from respite care to practical assistance like shopping. Counsellors are available to discuss all of the difficult emotional and social issues that can arise within families during this challenging time.

Hospice staff work closely with a range of health care providers so at no point in time is a patient locked into any specific place of care. If the need was felt for in-patient care there are facilities within hospitals, or as independent units, to which the patient can be referred. This may at times include returning, if needed, to the curative hospital system. Flexibility and a commitment to listening to the needs of the patient and their family determine the planning for such referrals. In short, hospices provide many solutions tailored to the specific needs of patients and their carers.

Hospice staff are used to anticipating needs, providing early notice to patients and their carers of expected changes, and being there with assistance when such changes occur. This is all done with the goodwill of active listening, warmth and compassion. Understandably, it is common for those touched by the hospice experience to learn with surprise that they were able to cope with a situation they thought was originally beyond their capacities.

Although many have a strong preference for being cared for at home, there are other valued in-patient options for those who wish to choose otherwise.

Timely referrals

There are a lot of pressures within mainstream health care (the term is call the 'technological imperative') that mean that individuals can be inappropriately treated with invasive, hi-tech interventions right to the end. This process can rob families of important quality time and can make it difficult for them to explore other alternatives as they feel guilty if they do not follow through on every offer to treat. In such a system referral to hospice will not be made until it is too late.

Ample time is needed to build relationships with hospice staff and to gain knowledge and confidence in the process. As the hospice emphasis is on the quality of living it is important to have the time to talk, to laugh, to reflect and to share meaningful experiences. Consequently, the earlier contact is made the better. In the present system timely referrals are not likely to happen so it usually takes persistence on the part of the family to make sure the appropriate contacts and arrangements are made. All efforts in this regard will be well rewarded because hospice care not only provides a gentle, respectful experience for the patient, but also leaves the family feeling nourished, supported and cared for.

The choice is yours

Individuals and their families coping with haematological malignancies, as much as anyone else, require the caring, respect and quality of life that the hospice experience has to offer. It is important that you know that this alternative exists. Informed consent and respect for the individual's autonomy are now ethically and legally enshrined in our health care system. So you not only should be routinely given information on the hospice alternative but have every right to insist on a timely and appropriate referral.

Appendix 1

WHAT ARE THEY TALKING ABOUT?

Most commonly newly diagnosed individuals and their families feel disorientated and intimidated when confronted by the unfamiliar medical world of haematological malignancy. The complicated technical language and complex medical processes can make the hospital setting seem like an alien space inhabited by experts who talk another language and who have sophisticated knowledge beyond the powers of comprehension of ordinary folks. Most will be entering this world in a state of shock from being confronted with a serious diagnosis and for many this will all be happening away from the comfort of their home town or familiar medical centre. This will be happening in the high-tech world of the specialist metropolitan treatment hospital.

Many will be driven by their sense of mastery and will take up the challenge to absorb and understand in great detail the offerings of this knowledge base. Such individuals will immediately access the Internet or the local medical library for information. Others, although they try, will be too numb to function and even with all the will in the world will not be in the emotional space to absorb such information. Still others will react with a strong sense of withdrawal only seeking enough facts to allow them to comply with the suggested treatment routine.

If you are in the early stages try not to be frightened about being overwhelmed as it will be no time at all before you will be conversing with sophistication. People quickly absorb both the ideas and the language and to their family and friends will eventually sound as bewildering as the experts. Indeed, one of the problems reported by those who return to homes located away from the metropolitan specialist hospitals is that their knowledge of the disease and its treatments is so far ahead of their local health care professionals. The absorption of this knowledge, similar to the process of learning any language, will be gradual and not necessarily with the individual aware of the progress they are making.

As with every aspect of coping with these illnesses there is no golden mean or level of knowledge that is essential for coping. Each individual will absorb the information at their own rate, according to their own need to know and prior understanding of medical concepts. In the best of worlds there should be a fit between your need to know and the provision of information by the health professionals who care for you. Unfortunately, all hospitals are very busy places and there is now ample evidence that, even where there is the best of intentions, individuals do not receive enough information for their needs. The reality is that to a large degree the responsibility still rests on the shoulders of the patient and their loved ones to assert their need for information. This will not be easy in a medical system where you only have the attention of your doctor for a brief time and feel somewhat intimidated in the hospital setting. Most people find that writing a list of questions before the meeting with the doctor helps them remember what to ask. It is now known that during initial interviews it is essential for the patient to be accompanied by a carer because the emotional reaction to being told about the diagnosis will, for most, block out their capacity to absorb information.

Following is an introductory summary and overview of the basic medical concepts informing diagnosis and treatment. It is not only designed for those just starting out in treatment, but also for those who wish to consult a reference at various times throughout treatment.

The intent underpinning this written discussion of clinical information is to provide the reader with a solid introductory baseline of information and a working knowledge for functioning in the area. However, it can only act as a starting point for gathering information. The golden rule for understanding information on haematological malignancies is that circumstances alter cases. Only a detailed medical consultation will provide the exact facts of each individual's case. In no way can the information contained in this text replace the open exchange of information you will need to develop with the health professionals who care for you or your loved one.

As this is clinical/scientific information the liberty has been taken of referencing each fact provided. In this way interested readers can go to the source for further information. The process of referencing was also undertaken to assure readers that the information that has been provided has been validated by a rigorous process of scientific peer review.

Haematological malignancies and related disorders cover a wide range of diagnostic groups and they all have defining characteristics and separate treatment protocols. Consequently, after the brief introduction to this area, each diagnostic group will be discussed separately.

What diagnostic group is that?
The Leukaemias

The word cancer, derived from the word *canker* a name for a 'eating, spreading sore or ulcer', refers to diseases that have in common the uncontrolled growth of cells.[12] Cancer begins when a cell breaks free from the normal restraints on uncontrolled growth and spreads.[18] The word leukaemia literally means 'white blood' because in the case of these diseases it is the altered white blood cells that multiply rapidly.[12]

Although popularly thought of as a disease of the blood, leukaemia is actually a cancer of the blood forming organs and the bone marrow.[11,12,20] Consequently, to understand leukaemia and related haematological diseases it is important to know a little about the formation and function of the blood. Blood, the sticky red fluid that circulates round the body in system of blood vessels, is the transport system for carrying life sustaining substances from one part of the body to another.[12] The blood supplies food, oxygen, hormones, and other chemicals to all of the body's cells.[20] It helps remove waste products and assists the lymph system in fighting infection.[20] The whole blood is composed of red cells (*erythrocytes*), the white blood cells (*leukocytes*) and the platelets that circulate in a clear straw coloured fluid known as *plasma*.[12,20] It may help to understand the importance of the role of the marrow in producing blood cells to know that at any point in time there are an estimated three million red blood cells and one hundred and twenty thousand white blood cells being produced every second.[12]

The production of blood cells (known as *haematopoiesis*) begins with the formation of immature cells (known as *stem cells*) in the bone marrow, the spongy interior of the large bones.[12,20] Each stem cell is highly active, producing as many as thousands of cells daily.[20] When the blood is healthy the numbers of circulating cells (red, white and platelets) is kept in balance and worn out cells are routinely removed.[20]

Although all of the blood cells come from the same original cell (called a *stem* or *precursor* cell), they quickly divide into two major families (the *myeloid* and the *lymphoid* families) and into a number of different types of blood cells within these families.[20] There is a range of different types of leukaemias depending on the type of cells affected by the disease.[14,20]

All forms are considered treatable and some are potentially curable, and the approaches to treatment are evolving steadily.[4]

In common with all of the haematological malignancies, the leukaemias are not contagious and cannot be passed on from the patient to others.[23]

The Myeloid Family

The myeloid family includes all of the red blood cells, platelets and a number of the white blood cells. These cells carry out the following functions in maintaining a healthy body:

- The function of red blood cells (*erythrocytes*) is to transport the oxygen (the fuel for energy) from the lungs to all tissues of the body[20] If there is a shortage of red blood cells the individual will feel tired and 'run-down'.[12]
- Platelets help prevent excessive bleeding by forming clots at

injured sites.[20] They stop the body from bleeding when it is cut or bruised by sticking together to form a 'plug' at the site of the damaged blood vessel.[12]

- White cells are the body's defence system and help to fight infection and disease.[20] There are three major groups of mature white blood cells (*leukocytes*), two of which are the white cells of the myeloid family (the *granulocytes* or *monocytes*), found mainly in the blood.[20] The granulocytes are further subdivided into eosinophils, basophils, and neutrophils.[20] A decrease in neutrophils is called neutropenia, which may result in an increased susceptibility to infections and ulcerations of the mucous membranes.[20]

When leukaemia affects cells in this family it is called myeloid, myelocytic, myelogenous, or granulocytic leukaemia.[20]

The Lymphoid Family

The cells of the lymphoid family are white cells that are not just found in the blood, but heavily populate the lymphatic system.[12] The *lymphatic system*, a body-wide arrangement of tiny drainage channels, is also involved in defending the body against infection and disease.[12] The lymphoid white cells (known as *lymphocytes*) circulate in a fluid (known as *lymph*) in tissue throughout the body including the lymph glands, the liver, and the spleen.[20] The lymph nodes or lymphatic glands, the filter system for the lymph, are packed with lymphocytes and during infection become swollen.[12]

There are two significant types of lymphocytes, T cell and B cells, and each provide a different type of immunity.[12,20] When leukaemia affects the cells from this family it is called lympho-blastic, lymphoid, lymphocytic, or lymphatic leukaemia.[20]

Types of Leukaemia

The leukaemias are classified into either *myeloid* or *lymphoid* depending on the family of cells affected.[14] These groups are further subdivided depending on the degree of maturation of the proliferating cells.[14] Hence, within these groups there can be either an *acute* form (rapidly progressing without treatment), or a *chronic* form (slower progression) where the damage to the cell formation happens in the later stage of cell development.[12,14] There are thus four common groups:

- *Acute Lymphoblastic Leukaemia (ALL)* – This disease can also be referred to as Acute Lymphocytic Leukaemia or Acute Lymphatic Leukaemia, and in turn can be classified into three different sub-groups.[20] ALL is the most common type of leukaemia in children, accounting for approximately 80 to 85 per cent of cases, whereas in adults only approximately 20 per cent of cases of acute leukaemias are ALL.[14,20] In adults, it is relatively rare.[16,20] The diagnosis is made from blood and marrow films which show the presence of a great number of abnormal (immature) white cells (Lymphocytes) in blood that has reduced numbers of other types of normal cells.[1,14] As a rule of thumb, the marrow must show over 30 per cent of blasts.[1] The large numbers of circulating abnormal cells can be seen by the fact that normal blood has less than 5 per cent of the young Lymphocytes (known as *blast cells*) where as during the disease this may increase to 50–95 per cent.[20] Presenting signs and symptoms are usually related to low blood counts including lethargy, bruising, malaise, fever, and infection.[14] Although decades ago this disease was quickly lethal, modern treatments now aim for either complete remission or possible cure.[34] Poor prognosis is indicated by factors which include: age over 40 years, the presence of the *Philadelphia Chromosome* (Ph'+ve), or T or B cell sub-types.[1,13,15,16] There are several stages in treatment. The first is *remission induction* (strategies to totally reduce the number of leukaemic cells) and is usually more intense with adults.[1,15] The second, *consolidation therapy,* is treatment given to further reduce the number of remaining cells.[1,15] Consolidation therapy is administered at a relatively high level of intensity to patients already in complete remission.[15] Prior to beginning this phase of therapy, patients have normal blood counts and generally a good performance status, as the *consolidation therapy* is used to 'mop up' residual leukaemic cells and lessen the risk of relapse.[4,15] This is followed by *maintenance therapy*, which is low level therapy which can last for up to two to three years and aims to keep the disease in remission and ensure the body eliminates remaining cells.[15,16] Treatment strategies are also directed, concurrently with systemic chemotherapy, at preventing the disease from entering the Central Nervous System (known as *CNS Prophylaxis*).[15,16] This involves the administration of drugs into the cerebrospinal fluid of the spinal cord as the CNS remains a sanctuary site and without treatment a sub-set of patients will develop CNS disease.[15,16] The other so-called sanctuary site is the testicles.[16] The disease can relapse and when this occurs the remission can become increasingly more difficult and patients can become resistant to the drugs previously used.[15] Cytotoxics used in current induction regimens are commonly known as the 'four drugs' (vincristine, prednisone, anthracycline, and cyclophosphamide or asparaginase) or the 'five drugs' (vincristine, prednisone, anthracycline, cyclophosphamide, and asparaginase).[15] Drugs used in consolidation therapy can include cytarabine (Ara-C) combined with other drugs, most typically anthracyclines, epidophillotoxins, or antimetabolites (such as methotrexate).[15] For some patients at risk of relapse BMT will be offered during first remission to provide an improved chance of long-term cure.[15,16]

• *Chronic Lymphoblastic Leukaemia (CLL)* – This is the most common form of leukaemia.[15,20] It is diagnosed by an excess of *lymphocytes* in the blood.[20] CLL is rare below the age of 40 years, and the incidence increases with age, and mainly affects elderly people.[1,20] CLL cannot be cured and treatment is designed to relieve symptoms.[1,4,15] It usually involves the build-up of diseased white cells, usually of the B cell variety (95 per cent). Although in a small number of cases (5 per cent) will involve the T cells indicating a more aggressive disease.[1,13,15] In over 25 per cent of patients the disease is indolent and they will have no symptoms at the time of diagnosis, so may not be offered treatment.[1,13]

Others will only require monitoring of their disease (observation phase) with attention given to avoiding and treating infections.[13] On those occasions when the patient is extremely sick at the time of initial diagnosis, appropriate therapy is instituted without undue delay.[13] In this form of leukaemia the white cells (*lymphocytes*) accumulate in the blood, bone marrow, lymph nodes and spleen, because of the cell's inability to die as normally such cells would be programmed to do.[15] For some, this process can eventually lead to pressure in these organs which will interrupt the normal production blood cells.[15] Consequently, these patients may eventually experience symptoms requiring treatment such as unexplained fever, fatigue (from low red cell count), frequent infections (low mature white cell count), weight loss, sweats, shortness of breath, pain from the spleen, and the risk of bleeding (low platelet count).[1,4,13] Sometimes a patient feels uneasy and self-conscious from a cosmetic consideration when masses of lymph nodes are easily visible.[13] The prognosis for CLL depends on the extent of disease at presentation.[4] In a small number of patients the disease may evolve to a more aggressive form known as *lymphoma* or *prolymphocytic leukaemia*.[13] Available treatments typically involve the *alkylating agents*, such as *cyclophosphamide* and *chlorambucil*, at times accompanied by prednisone,[1,15] or the *designer drugs* such as *fludarabine* or *CDA*.[13] The treatment is continued until the symptoms and signs of the disease have regressed to a considerable extent.[1] Many patients with CLL live for long periods of time without requiring therapeutic intervention. The ability to identify such patients has improved in recent years.[15]

- *Acute Myelogenous Leukaemia (AML)* – Also known as Acute Granulocytic Leukaemia or Acute Myelocytic Leukaemia.[20] Although this disease affects the myeloid cells (white cells such as granulocytes, monocytes, red blood cells and platelets) it particularly affects one form of the white cells (infection fighters) called the granulocytes.[14] The development of these cells goes wrong and there become too many immature cells that can eventually start to block the blood vessels. Although occurring in children and adolescents it is more common in older people and those who have previously had chemotherapy.[15,16] It is the most common form of acute leukaemia in adults.[20] Although it is possible for the condition to be diagnosed in patients with no symptoms (perhaps as a result of a routine check-up) the symptoms are usually similar to most leukaemias including the side effects of anaemia (pallor and tiredness), bone pain, problems with bleeding or problems with infections.[1,15] The diagnosis is confirmed by the presence of a great number of immature (blast cells) myeloid cells when the patient's blood is examined under the microscope.[14] The basic requirement for a diagnosis of AML is the presence of 30 per cent or more blasts in the blood or bone marrow.[14] Standard induction therapy is based on the combination of cytarabine with an anthracycline.[15] The patient's age is crucial in relation to treatment in AML.[9,15] The likelihood of initial disease remission and of remaining in complete remission (CR) declines with age.[9,15] If the patient relapses, a second remission may be more difficult to obtain than the first.[15]

- *Chronic Myeloid Leukaemia (CML)* – This disease can occur at any age, although it is commoner in middle and old age.[1] CML is diagnosed by genetic tests that establish the presence of what is known as the *Philadelphia (Ph')Chromosome*.[1,4,13] Initially the patient may not have symptoms and the condition may only be diagnosed through a routine blood count.[1] During the chronic stage of this disease symptoms can be managed through the judicious use of chemotherapy (including drugs such as *Busulphan, Hydroxyurea,* and *Interferon*) and the individual can feel well for many years.[1,4,15] The disease can undergo a *transformative stage* where it transforms into a more malignant variety of leukaemia (usually AML but for a smaller number ALL) requiring more intensive therapy.[1,13] The transformation is usually accompanied by malaise, enlarged spleen, bone pain and an increasing number of immature white cells (know as *blast cells*) and the prognosis is not good.[4,13]

Because the *acute* leukaemia affects the cells in the very early stage of life, thus stopping the cells from functioning at all, the patient usually requires immediate treatment.[20] In contrast, the *chronic* forms affect mature cells which are able to maintain much of their normal function and so do not always require immediate treatment.[20]

The diagnostic tests for leukaemia include a blood test and a combination of bone marrow tests (*aspiration* and *biopsy*).[12] A blood test may show low haemoglobin, low levels of normal white cells, and low platelet count as well as high numbers of leukaemic blast cells.[20] The *aspiration* involves pushing a needle into the marrow to remove a few drops of fluid which is smeared onto a microscope slide and examined to determine cell types.[12] The biopsy involves removing, by a specially designed marrow coring needle, a small cylindrical core of bone together with bone marrow about the size of thin spaghetti. The sample for the bone marrow obtained from the biopsy is microscopically examined to determine the diagnostic group.[12] The two methods are complementary. Other tests include examining the chromosomes of the marrow sample cells or testing with chemical reagents. All help to establish the diagnosis and classification.[12]

* *Childhood Leukaemia* – For definitional purposes, childhood refers to children below the age of 15 years.[1,6] Because this is a special area, and exciting in terms of the recent progress in treatment outcomes, it will be dealt with separately here. Leukaemia is the most common form of childhood cancer, and ALL accounts for 80 per cent of all cases, AML and its variants for 17 per cent of the remainder.[1,12] It should be noted however, that leukaemia is still rare with estimation being that in the first fifteen years of life the odds of developing leukaemia are less than one in 1500.[12] Although much of the information with regards to leukaemia has already covered in the above discussion, it needs to be clearly stated that childhood ALL has different clinical features and a much better prognosis than adult ALL or AML at any age.[1,35] Indeed, childhood ALL has provided a landmark in cancer therapy as the first disseminated and other-

wise lethal malignancy to be curable in the majority of patients.[6,35] ALL usually presents at 4-5 years, after a few weeks of malaise, pallor, mouth ulcers, bone pains, sometimes *petechiae* (small spots of red or purple found on the skin) and perhaps a fever even in the absence of obvious infection.[1,12] Clinical signs can include a deficiency of red cells (anaemia), a shortage of platelets (thrombocytopenia), enlarged lymph nodes, elevated white cell count.[1] Survival in ALL is better in girls than in boys.[1] A standard protocol for ALL will progress along the following well established phases. The first stage, which lasts for 3-4 weeks, is *remission induction* in which intense chemotherapy (using drugs such as *vincristine, pred-nisolone, asparaginase,* and *doxorubicin*) is given to totally reduce the number of leukaemic cells.[1,6,27] The second stage (called *consolidation*) involves further intensive treatment (using drugs such as *asparaginase* and *methotrexate*) where the disease cells are further reduced.[1,6,27] Thirdly, treatment (called *central nervous system treatment*) is given in spaces such as the brain and spinal cord where chemotherapy does not penetrate to prevent relapses by ensuring that the leukaemia cells are killed in these spaces.[1,6] Strategies used are lumbar punctures, and high doses of intravenous drugs (for example *Methotrexate*) or cranial irradiation. The fourth stage, which usually last for about 2 years, is *maintenance* (also known as *continuing*) chemotherapy (usually *methotrexate, vincristine,* and *pred-nisolone*) and aims to completely destroy any remaining cancer cells.[1,6] It has been well known for many years that the testes represent a site of extramedullary leukaemia for boys with ALL and strategies to address this are built into many protocols.[27] During treatment the child is at risk of infection, particularly with viral infections such as measles and chicken pox, because of the low white cell counts.[27] It is standard practice to stop treatment of children with ALL who have been in remission for 2-3 years.[27] Relapse is considered unusual beyond 1 year after treatment has stopped.[1] The risk of relapse decreases with increasing time off therapy, and children who have no return of the disease with no treatment after 4-5 years have a good chance of being cured for life.[19] Some children do relapse.[19] This is serious during treatment, but if following treatment then further intensive treatment can lead to a long term second remission.[1,27] Bone marrow transplants may also be offered as a treatment option.[27] Relapses rarely occur in children who are off treatment for several years.[19]

There are differences between the treatments and outcomes of ALL and AML.[35] In comparison to childhood ALL, paediatric AML has been more difficult to eradicate with conventional treatment programs.[36] The children are sometimes offered a BMT, either autologous or allogeneic, after an initial period of intensive chemotherapy.[35]

Childhood leukaemia is not infectious and it is not possible for one child to 'catch' leukaemia from another.[23] The cause of childhood leukaemia is still unknown.[23] The aim of treatment for all acute leukaemias is now for cure.[6]

- *Other Childhood Haematological Disorders* – Non-Hodgkin's lymphomas are rather more common in childhood than Hodgkin's disease and are the third most frequent childhood cancer.[1] The majority of NHL in childhood are B cell tumours.[1]

The Related Blood Diseases

There are a number of related diseases that involve either the myeloid or lymphoid cells. The present discussion will provide a short overview of the most common of these diseases.

The Lymphomas

Lymphomas are cancers of the complex network of specialised organs and cells, collectively known as the immune system, that defends the body against infection.[20] The organs of the immune system are often referred to as 'lymphatic' organs as they are concerned with the growth, development, and circulation of the lymphocytes (white cells) used in the body's defence against infection and disease.[20] The lymphatic organs include the bone marrow, thymus, spleen, lymph nodes, as well as the tonsils, and appendix.[20] Lymphatic vessels carry lymph, a fluid containing white blood cells, to all parts of the body.[20] In all forms of lymphoma, the cells in the lymph tissue begin growing abnormally and, if left untreated, spread to other organs.[20]

The two main forms of Lymphomas are Hodgkin's Disease and non-Hodgkin's Lymphoma.[20] In both groups of the disease the first sign is usually a swelling of the lymph glands, commonly in the neck, armpit or groin.[20] Most of the symptoms are present in other illness and the only sure way to determine the diagnosis is by a biopsy (examining under the microscope in a laboratory a sample of the cells taken from an affected node).[20]

Hodgkin's Disease (HD)

In recent decades the prognosis of this disease has greatly improved, both for patients with localised disease who are often curable by radiotherapy, and for those with disseminated disease treated with chemotherapy drugs.[1] Most people with HD, no matter what the sub-type, can now be cured.[1,20] The best chance of cure is when the patient first presents with the disease, as recurrence of disease usually worsens the outlook.[1,20]

HD most often arises in lymph nodes, usually in the chest or neck.[15,16] Most patients accidentally notice an enlarged, painless lymph node in the neck or elsewhere, and HD is diagnosed through a biopsy.[1,15] Symptoms include weight loss, fever, night sweats, fatigue, and sometimes infections because of altered immune function.[1,14,16] The most common age for onset of the disease is either between 10 and 20 years or over 50 years, reaching a maximum at 70 years and over.[1]

HD is recognised diagnostically by the presence of a particular type of cell, found in the lymph nodes of the patient, called the Reed-Sternberg cell.[1,14,16] The clinical picture of individuals with this disease can vary depending on which of the sub-types of the disease they have.[1,15] The most common form of classification (known as the *Lukes-Butler*

Scheme) depends on the microscopic appearance of the cells (histological classification) taken during a biopsy.[15,1] Tests can also be done to stage the disease (that is, document its spread throughout the body) and staging classifications vary from Stage I to IV.[1,16]

The treatments usually include radiation for the early stages, with combination chemotherapy for later stage disease.[1,15,16] Combination drug therapy can include programs such as MOPP (Nitrogen mustard, Vincristine, Procarbazine, Prednisone), ChlVPP (Chlorambucil, Vinblastine, Procarbazine, Prednisone) or ABVD (Doxorubicin, Bleomycin, Vinblastine, Dacarbazine).[15,20] Short courses of steroids can be administered. Bone Marrow Transplantation can be offered to patients who are experiencing relapse or drug-resistant disease.[1]

Non-Hodgkin's Lymphoma (NHL)

These malignancies of lymph cells can be found either in the lymph glands or in any soft tissue of the body and are much more common than HD. [15] Because of the young average age of lymphoma patients and the resulting number of years of life lost to these diseases, NHL are considered very important group of diseases.[15] The incidence of NHL is rising, with the disease is usually found in older people, although there are a number of rare forms found in childhood or young adults.[1,15] The first symptom can be a painless swelling of the lymph node in the neck, groin, armpits or elsewhere in the body, usually associated with a degree of lethargy.[16] Other signs of the disease can include persistent fever, severe night sweats, persistent tiredness, or unexplained weight loss or generalised itchy skin.[16]

There is a broad range of NHL and the type of lymphocyte involved usually determines the type of lymphoma.[15] Doctors confirm the diagnosis through an examination of cells of the enlarged lymph gland under the microscope.[16] The literature acknowledges that there is a 'bewildering profusion of terminology' to describe the different types of non-Hodgkin's lymphomas.[1] Non-Hodgkin's lymphomas are also graded (low grade, intermediate grade, high-grade).[1]

Combination chemotherapy is the treatment of choice in all patients irrespective of tumour stage.[16] Radiotherapy may be used to treat sites of prior bulk disease on completion of the course of chemotherapy.[16]

There are rare types of aggressive forms of non-Hodgkin's lymphomas (*Lymphoblastic Lymphoma* and *Burkitt's Lymphoma*) which grow rapidly.[20]

Multiple Myeloma (MM)

MM is mainly a disease of the elderly, rare in people under 40 years old, and is more likely to occur in males.[1,16] Myeloma is not a curable disease.[16] Known risk factors include exposure to radiation, either a single high dose or chronic low dose exposure.[16,21] Agricultural workers who are exposed to pesticides also have a higher incidence.[21] In this disease the very mature lymphoid cells, called *plasma cells*, build up in the body especially in the cavities of the bone marrow and which can occasionally be found in the blood.[1] There is an infiltration of both the bone and the bone marrow by malignant plasma cells, and the infiltration is often patchy (that is in many sites) and hence the name multiple myeloma.[1] Any bone can be affected and common sites include vertebrae, pelvis, skull, ribs and proximal long bones.[1] The symptoms include bone pain because of the pressure of the massing of plasma cells in the cavity of the bones.[16] This cell pressure can eventually undermine the production of cells for the blood and can lead to the destruction of the bones themselves.[1]

The disease can be present for several years before the tumour has expanded sufficiently to cause symptoms.[1] Symptoms of MM can include weakness/fatigue, bone pain, nausea, clouded consciousness (headache; blurred vision), recurrent infections, and anorexia (due to hypercalcaemia), and anaemia.[1,16,21] The pain is usually dull or aching, often felt in the spine, ribs or pelvis.[1] Pathological bone fractures are common and acute back pain from a crushed vertebra is often the initial symptom noted.[1] Also, the immune system will be damaged with a reduced capacity to fight infection.[1] The kidneys can be overloaded and become affected.[1]

Multiple Myeloma is diagnosed by the presence of a protein (known as the *Bence-Jones protein*) in the urine which is a by-product of antibody of the cancerous plasma cell.[1] The protein is detected by immunoelectrophoresis of the urine.[1] The diagnosis is further confirmed by evidence of increased numbers of abnormal plasma cells and evidence of bone damage.[21] Where the bone damage is quite extensive there may be increased levels of calcium in the blood (known as *hypercalcaemia*) which is associated with loss of appetite, nausea, vomiting, dehydration and constipation.[1]

Most patients (90 per cent) are symptomatic at diagnosis requiring treatment.[21] Combinations of alkylating agent melphalan and prednisolone given orally are used and stopped when the patient reaches stability (known as the plateau phase).[16,1] During the plateau phase no further response is seen despite continued treatment.[21] This phase may last for some time but relapse is inevitable.[21] Radiotherapy is often required as part of the initial treatment, particularly with patients that have painful bone deposits in the vertebrae or long bones, especially if at risk of pathological fracture or cord compression.[1] Bone marrow and peripheral stem cell transplants are now offered as a treatment option. [21] Although the side effects are difficult for many patients to handle, the drug *interferon* has also been found to have some beneficial affect on slowing the progression of the disease.[21]

Aplastic Anaemia

This is a form of anaemia that is characterised by defective function of the blood-forming organs (such as the bone marrow).[30] When the marrow fails to produce adequate numbers of cells the patient becomes anaemic, has a low white cell count (leucopenia) and a low platelet count (thrombocytopenia).[33] It is believed to be caused by toxic agents (such as chemicals, drugs or X-rays) or is of unknown (*idiopathic*) origin.[30,33] Patients present with lethargy and weakness due to anaemia, a tendency to bruise with undue ease due to loss of platelets, and less frequently, of an inability to overcome infections because of low white blood counts (*neutropenia*).[33] Pallor, purple spots on the skin (*purpura*) and less frequently, signs of infection are other indications of the disease.[33] Blood counts show all blood cells are reduced including red, white and platelets. [33] Bone marrow aspirates are also used diagnostically.[33] The management of the disease can be three fold. Firstly, a search for, and elimination of, the possible drug or chemical cause is undertaken. Secondly, supportive therapy, consisting of blood and platelet transfusions and antibiotics, are given when required. Thirdly, transplantation can be offered in some cases with successful outcome.[33]

Other Related Bone Marrow and Blood Diseases

There are a number of other malignant diseases associated with myeloid and lymphoid blood cells including:

- *Myelodysplastic syndromes (MDS)* – Although five disease types, classified according to the major abnormality present, are collected under the title of this syndrome precise categorisation may be difficult and arbitrary.[1] The incidence of MDS is difficult to define precisely because of the heterogeneity of the syndromes and the presence of benign types which often go untreated.[15] MD is rarely seen before 50 years of age but rapidly increases in incidence in older populations.[15,32] Usually an elderly patient presents with an anaemia which proves refractory to treatment with persistent low white cell count (*neutropenia*) and low platelet levels (*thrombocytopenia*).[32] Thus, the presenting symptoms are pallor, fatigue, fever, petechiae, bruising, or bleeding or an abnormal finding on a routine complete blood count.[15] Typically there is no enlargement of the liver, spleen or lymph nodes.[32] It is diagnosed histologically (an examination of the cells under the microscope) from a sample of marrow. MDS have an inherent tendency to progress to acute leukaemia and for this reason the syndromes were previously commonly called *pre-leukaemia* or *smouldering leukaemia*.[1,15] This defect is known to lead in a small number (approximately 20 per cent) to a form of leukaemia (Acute Myeloid Leukaemia), but there is no corresponding syndrome for ALL.[12,15] Some MDS are well defined and their course and outlook known, others are not always clear how they will progress.[12] Most MDS are treated with supportive measures directed at relieving symptoms only and chemotherapy is deferred until the development of overt acute leukaemia, if it occurs.[13] Alkylating agents and radiation therapy used in cancer treatments are implicated as causes of MD.[15]

* *Myeloproliferative Disorders (MPD)* – There are three diseases grouped together under the heading of this disorder that are characterised by the over-production of blood cells in the bone marrow.[13,33] In a small number of cases each of these diseases can develop into *acute myeloid leukaemia.*[13,14,27]

* *Polycythaemia Ruba Vera* – This rare condition is predominantly associated with an inappropriate increased number of circulating red blood cells, in the absence of an accompanying disease.[13,14] It is a disorder of older people.[33] It is attributed to abnormal activity of the bone marrow stem cells.[33] It is insidious in onset and symptoms may be present for several years before medical attention is sought.[13,27] The presenting symptoms relate to the increased red blood cells and include headache, weakness, blurred vision and dizziness.[14,27,33] There is a risk of blood clots which can be dangerous if lodged in the brain or heart.[14] Although there is no cure for this condition, it is considered benign.[13] There are treatments to relieve the symptoms such as taking amounts of the patient's blood on a regular basis to reduce the pressure of the red cells. In some cases drugs such as *hydroxyurea, interferon* can be useful.[13,27]

* *Essential Thrombocythaemia* – In this case the bone marrow produces too many platelets and these may not function as required causing either blood clots or bleeding problems.[13,27,33] Platelets in polycythaemia are often functionally abnormal.[33] Again treatments include aspirin to reduce the possibility of clots, or drugs such as *hydroxyurea* to reduce platelet counts.[27] In some cases procedures involving the direct removal of platelets from the blood (*platelet pheresis*) will be used but are only considered a stop gap measure.[13] Marrow depressants such as

busulphan, chlorambucil and cyclophosphamide can be used to damp down marrow production.[33]

• *Myelofibrosis* – This condition is characterised by an increase in fibres (known as *reticulin fibres*) in the bone marrow.[29,33] The invasion of fibres can scar up to 25 per cent of the marrow volume.[29,30] Because of the reduced effectiveness of the bone marrow the liver and spleen begin, not very effectively, to take over the function of cell production.[30] Consequently, the characteristics of the condition are decreased red blood cells (*anaemia*), enlarged spleen, immature blood cells in the circulation and cell production (*haematopoiesis*) occurring in the liver and spleen.[31] The classical presentation of this disease is of an older patient with a very large spleen.[33] Often they complain of loss of energy due to moderate anaemia, discomfort due to an enlarged spleen or to thrombotic complications (such as thrombosis in leg veins).[33]

• *Paroxysmal Nocturnal Haemoglobinuria (PNH)* – A rare condition that gets it name because the body excretes the red blood pigment (known as *haemoglobin*) in the urine typically at night, with excess in the urine (*Haemoglobinurea*) noted upon urination after awakening.[30] This breakdown of red blood cells is accompanied by a reduction in other blood cells (white cells and platelets) and is thus characterised by increase susceptibility to infection (*leukopenia*) and problems with bleeding (*thrombocytopenia*).[29,30]

• *Immune (Idiopathic) Thrombocytopenic Purpura (ITP)* – This condition is characterised by bleeding into the skin and other organs caused by deficiency of platelets.[31] ITP is a diagnosis of exclusion where the causes are unknown (*idiopathic*) and the diseases known to be associated with secondary shortage of platelets (*thrombocytopenia*) have been excluded.[29] The disorder is the result of accelerated platelet destruction attributed to an immunologic process.[29] Acute ITP, which is common, is a disease of children that may follow a viral infection.[31] It can last for a few weeks to a few months and usually has no residual effect.[31] The chronic form, which is rare, is more common in adolescents and adults, begins more insidiously and lasts longer.[29,31] It is more common in women with a three to one ratio of female to male.[29] Excessive bleeding (haemorrhage and bruisability) is the most common symptom, hence the name *Purpura* (purple colour or bruising under the skin), and the patient often has tiny red dots (known as *petechiae*) on the skin or mucous membranes.[29] The condition can be transient.[29] The efficacy of most treatments used in ITP is uncertain, especially in view of the possibility of spontaneous remission (80 per cent spontaneous remission).[29] Refractory ITP may respond to low dose corticosteroids or pulse high-dose dexamethasone, some forms of combination chemotherapy, or removal of spleen (*splenectomy*).[29]

- *Mast Cell Leukaemia (MCL)* – A mast cell is a large cell with numerous heparin-containing basophilic granules (basophils are types of white blood cells) that occur especially in the connective tissue.[30] These cells produce heparin.[30] MCL is a very rare form of acute leukaemia, characterised by increased numbers of mast cells in one or more tissues or organs, particularly in the skin.[29] Clinical features include fever, anorexia, weight loss, fatigue, abdominal colic, diarrhoea, bone pain and enlarged liver or spleen.[30]

- *Hairy Cell Leukaemia* – This is a very rare type of leukaemia, related to CLL, usually found in men and in the middle to older age group (50–70 years).[1,13] The diagnosis is indicated by a reduction of normal marrow cells (shown by a low red cell count, shortage of platelets, neutropenia) and the presence of 'hair-like' protrusions from the abnormal blood cells (abnormal mononuclear cells with irregular cytoplasmic projections) when examined under the microscope.[1,13] The presenting symptoms are often nonspecific and include fatigue, weakness, or abdominal discomfort.[15] On physical examination many patients have an enlarged spleen.[15] Drugs associated with treatment for this disease are *Chlorambucil* or *interferon* or *deoxycoformycin*.[1,13] The outlook for HCL is now considered to be very good with a number of effective treatments now available.

- *Plasma Cell Leukaemia* – This is a rare condition of the middle aged or elderly that needs to be distinguished from myeloma.[21] There are two principal types (*Primary and Secondary*). It is diagnosed as a primary disease when the peripheral blood contains 20 per cent circulating plasma cells.[21] Hypercalcaemia, renal failure and bony lesions are often present at diagnosis.[21] The disease has a particularly poor prognosis.[21]

- *Large Granular Lymphocytic Leukaemia* – A disease which usually runs a chronic benign course.[32] Patients with this very rare disease have chronic neutropenia and/or anaemia.[32] There are increased peripheral blood lymphocytes (type of white cell) which may be large and with a granular appearance.[32]

- *Monoclonal Gammopathy of Unknown Significance* – This is a rare condition, mainly found in older people, in which there is a high number of plasma proteins circulating in the blood.[1] When most of the protein being produced is one particular type this is called *monoclonal gammopathy*. When this cannot be attributed to disease (such as myeloma or lymphoma) it is labelled *of unknown significance*.[1] It is often found by chance on a routine check up. MGUS requires no treatment although in a small number it is seen to predispose to myeloma.[1]

- *Waldenstrom's Macro-globulinaemia* – Another disease which typically occurs in the elderley.[1] A rare chronic condition which has features in common with indolent non-Hodgkin's lymphoma and multiple myeloma (without the bone damage). The cells affected in this condition are the lymphocytes which produce an excess amount of antibody.[27] The diagnosis is made by the presence of cells typical for this disease (*lymphoplasma-cytoid*) and an abnormal amount of protein in the blood.[1] The most common symptoms include fatigue and bleeding.[27] There is often an enlargement of lymph nodes, liver and spleen, and patients can present with weakness, night-sweats, headache, mental confusion, retinal haemorrhages and renal impairment.[1] The disease is usually only slowly progressive and, in the absence of symptoms, treatment can be withheld.[1] Where treatment is given strategies such as *plasmapheresis* (the removal of some of the antibody from the blood using a machine), and chemotherapy (usually involving *chlorambucil* or *cyclophosphamide*) are employed.[1]

- *Amyloidosis* – This is a relatively rare condition as a clinically significant disease.[27] This is the term for a group of conditions in which an abnormal substance (called *amyloid*) is deposited in tissues throughout the body.[27] The production of this substance is quite common in the myelomas.[28] The symptoms usually involve weight loss, fatigue, kidney failure, and pain.[27] It is diagnosed by the presence of amyloid deposits found in tissue samples of the body.[27] Treatment is similar to that of multiple myeloma (involving drugs such as *melphalan* and *prednisolone*).[27]
- *Down's Syndrome and Leukaemia* – Leukaemia is twenty times more common in children with Down's Syndrome, particularly ALL and AML.[12]

Do we know the cause?

Most patients and their families, on receiving the diagnosis, will have very natural and understandable feelings of 'why me'. It is all too easy to take responsibility for the disease and suffer guilt for imagined avoidable causes. This experience of guilt can be exacerbated by the lack of information on cause. It often leads to a process of 'blaming the victim', a process where the patient and family not only have to cope with the misfortune of having to cope with these diseases but also, through ignorance, carry an unrealistic sense of responsibility for its causation. It is thus of utmost importance that all involved appreciate that conclusive statements on causation are not possible at this stage of our understanding of these diseases.

There is still a long way to go before medical science begins to understand the causes of these sets of diseases.[12,16,23] This short discussion will provide some data on the evidence that is presently available.

There is no evidence at all of these diseases being genetic in the sense of there being an obvious pattern of the diseases being inherited.[12,20,23]

Scientists have long known that retroviruses can cause leukaemias and lymphomas in certain animal species, but no such virus has been found in human cancer cells.[20] However, there is some evidence to suggest that Hodgkin's disease is at least in some age groups related to infection with Epstein-Barr virus (better known as the cause of glandular fever).[1,23] However, only a small number of people with the virus go on to develop Hodgkin's Disease.[23]

Tentative links are starting to be mapped with causative factors such as radiation. There is a well established risk factor of irradiation with Multiple Myeloma.[16] Also statistical evidence strongly suggests that ionising radiation, either from a single, large dose or repeated small doses, can induce leukaemia in humans.[20] However, many develop these diseases without exposure to the carcinogens.[12,13]

The link with power lines has not been established.[12]

ALL differs from most childhood diseases in being more prevalent in higher socio-economic groups.[23]

In Aplastic Anaemia there is some suggestion that certain drugs or chemicals (industrial and household) could be implicated in the illness. The risk of acute leukaemia is estimated to be 20 times higher for workers heavily exposed to benzene than for the general population.[20]

There is now conclusive evidence that in some cases the chemotherapy drugs used in treatment can at a later stage contribute to the development of secondary cancers.[20,25]

Appendix 2

TREATMENT INFORMATION

This chapter is designed to provide a brief overview of the principal concepts and technical terms in relation to the major treatment options in this area. The intent is to give the reader basic background information to assist with the challenging process of learning and understanding the 'language of treatment'.

Chemotherapy

Although the word chemotherapy refers to the use of any drugs or medications to treat diseases, today the term is usually associated with the administration of drugs as a method of cancer treatment. [20] The drugs used to kill cancer cells are called *cytotoxics* (which means toxic to cells). The aim of chemotherapy is not only to kill or shrink the primary tumour but also to kill metastasised cells.[16] All cells, both normal and cancer, go through phases of growth and development during their life cycle.[17] Chemotherapy drugs interfere with the cellular activities during one or more of these phases.[16,17]

The choice of anti-cancer drugs for each patient depends on the type and location of the cancer, its stage of development, how it affects normal body functions, and the general health of the patient. [20] In most cases chemotherapy is delivered in a dose which is calculated from the weight and height of the patient.[16] There are various ways these drugs can be administered, for example, by mouth (*orally* by tablet or capsule), by injection through the skin (*subcutaneous*), by injection through a vein (*intravenous*), by injection into a muscle (*intramuscular*), or through an implanted catheter or special line.[17]

These drugs usually circulate in the bloodstream to achieve a total body (*systemic*) effect.[20] It is standard practice now to administer a combination of drugs, which are commonly known by the first letters of the drugs included in the regimen.[16] The reason for this is twofold. Firstly, the different drugs exert different effects through different mechanisms and at different stages of the cell cycle. Secondly, combining drugs decreases the chance of drug resistance developing.[16] The goal of combination chemotherapy is to select drugs that are additive in therapy and sub-additive in toxicity.[17] Chemotherapy is delivered intermittently rather than at a constant low dose, to exploit the fact that malignant cells have a less effective repair capacity than normal cells.[16] They are usually given in cycles, with the next treatment given when the normal stem cells have had adequate time to recover from the last. If it is too soon the normal cells will suffer unacceptable toxicity and it is too late the cancer cells will be allowed to recover to their pre-treatment size and expand.[16] The length and frequency of chemotherapy will depend on the kind of cancer, the drugs being used and how the patient's body responds to them.[20] Drugs are usually administered daily, weekly, or monthly.[20] Sometimes treatment is given in an on-and-off cycle that includes rest periods so that the body has a chance to build healthy new cells and regain strength.[20]

One of the major problems with chemotherapy is that as well as killing the cancer cells it also kills the normal cells in the body.[17] The side effects will depend on the normal cells affected, with those most likely to be affected in the bone marrow, gastrointestinal tract, reproductive system, and hair follicles.[20,25] Thus, the side effects reported most often are myelosuppression, nausea and vomiting, anorexia, diarrhoea, fatigue, and hair loss.[20,25] Less frequently, organ systems (such as the kidneys, heart, nerves, lives and reproductive system) can be affected.[25] The drugs can also cause psychological alterations, such as anxiety and depression.[25] There is a great variation in the difference between the side effects experienced by individuals. It is important that patients are issued with a typed information sheet detailing the expected side-effects of treatment and are given the opportunity to ask questions and discuss their anxieties before they start chemotherapy.[16]

The patient's white cell count can be affected by chemotherapy thus leaving the individual vulnerable to infection during treatment.[22] The acute immunosuppressive effects of most drugs used in chemotherapy do not extend for prolonged periods beyond the time of active drug administration.[22] A very low white cell count is known as neutropenia and is strictly defined as a polymorphonuclear neutrophil count of $<0.5 \times 10^9$/L.[16] The blood count is at its lowest 10–14 days following treatment with chemotherapy.[16] One of the main symptoms of infections is a high temperature and most patients will be told to contact their doctor immediately if they have a high temperature as antibiotics will be required.

Other short-term effects can include nausea and vomiting, constipation, diarrhoea, tiredness, and soreness of the mouth (mucositis).[16] Hair loss (alopecia) results from a direct cytotoxic effect on dividing cells within hair follicles, and usually commences two weeks after treatment has been started.[16] Hair loss is almost always reversible.[22] Depending on the drugs used some patients can experience a tingling sensation and weakness in their hands and feet that may last for several months.[16] Each drug will be responsible for different side effects and so the treating hospital will provide patients with written information on the exact expected side-effects from the particular drugs used.

There are now strategies for combating side effects such as anti-nausea drugs (*anti-emetics*), adjustments in diets, mouth washes and mouth care strategies, avoidance of crowds and infections, antibodies for infections, platelets to prevent bleeding, blood transfusions to build red cell count, creams and lotions for dry or itchy skin, the provision of wigs for the time during the regrowth of hair loss and sperm banking and egg storage for infertility.[20] Drugs are now given (known as *growth factors*) to accelerate the body's recovery of blood cell production. Hair regrowth usually starts around two months after completion of treatment.[16]

Chemotherapy can be associated with long term problems such as infertility.[16] The cytotoxics used are also now known in some cases to produce secondary malignancies years later.[16] The drugs associated with carcinogenicity include Chlorambucil, Cyclophosphamide, Etoposide, Melphalan, Nitrogen mustard, Procarbazine.[16]

Radiation

Ionising radiation is a highly potent cytotoxic agent, (that is an agent used to kill cancer cells).[16] Radiation at high levels (for example, tens of thousands of times the amount used in X-rays) destroys the ability of cells to grow and divide.[20] Both normal and diseased cells are affected, but most normal cells are able to recover quickly.[20] It is this differential repair capacity that is exploited in radiotherapy.[16] By carefully aiming and timing the high-energy rays, doctors use radiation as an effective tool in cancer treatment.[20]

The treatment is usually administered by a radiologist (or radiation oncologist) in the radiotherapy department of the treating hospital, either as outpatient or inpatient.[20] The various machines that direct radiation to the cancer work in slightly different ways, as some are better for treating cancer near the skin surface and others work on sites deeper in the body.[20] Methods of administration allow for the prescription of precise doses of radiation to be delivered to the tumour.[16] The number of sessions and doses of radiation will depend on factors such as the type of disease and the size of the tumour mass.[20] After taking the patient's medical history the radiation oncologist will need X-rays or other tests to pinpoint the location and size of the cancer. In a process called *simulation* (using a machine called a *simulator*) the patient will be asked to lie very still on a table while the technologist uses a special machine to X-ray the cancer.[20] Removable ink marks will be placed on the skin to indicate the areas to be irradiated.[20] It is important for the patient to remain very still during treatment so that the radiation reaches only the area where it is needed.[20] The patient will not see or hear the radiation and, apart from a possible feeling of warmth or tingling in the area being treated, will not feel discomfort.[20]

Radiation can be accompanied by side effects such as general fatigue, skin problems, loss of appetite, nausea, and perhaps hair loss in the area being treated.[20] The side effects suffered will depend on the location of the site in the body where the radiation is given, for example radiation in the lower abdomen may lead to upset stomach or diarrhoea.[20] Radiation therapy in any part of the pelvis can create side effects in the reproductive system.[20] There is also some evidence that radiation can create secondary cancers many years after treatment.[15]

Radiotherapy may be administered with radical or palliative intent.[16] In cases of advanced disease, when a cure of the cancer is not likely, radiation therapy can still bring a large measure of relief.[20] The maximum dose that can be administered with 'acceptable' toxicity is given in radical radiotherapy. In palliative radiotherapy the total dose is not so important as symptom relief as the emphasis is on minimising side-effects of radiation.[16]

Patients undergoing radiotherapy do not become radioactive and are not a risk to others, including children.

Supportive Care

High-dose therapy requires intensive medical and nursing care.[5] Many of the drugs now used to combat leukaemia injure normal cells as well as cancer cells, so managing chemotherapy's side effects is an important part of treatment.[20] There are many interventions provided during treatment to ensure that the patient's body system is supported or bolstered whilst it is trying to cope with the onslaught of the intensive and toxic treatments.[4] Indeed, as many of the same drugs have been used for many years, the improved rates of remission are partly attributed to the developments in supportive care.[9] The focus of the care is the management of side effects, monitoring of toxicities, and prevention of complications.[5]

During the intensive stage blood products support is essential.[1] Platelets are given to prevent haemorrhaging and the infusion of red cells reduces the side effects of anaemia.[1,20] Steps, such as strict regimens for hand washing and dental hygiene, the provision of broad-spectrum antibiotics, and the cleaning and cooking of food, are taken to prevent or treat infections during the vulnerable time when the patient's immune system is suppressed because of the disease and treatment.[1,20] Patients are usually hospitalised and nursed in isolation during periods of profound neutropenia (reduction of white cells responsible for fighting infection).[4] Aggressive antibiotic therapy has greatly aided the treatment of infectious complications.[20] A semi-permanent in-dwelling central venous catheter (for example the Hickman catheter) will be inserted to help the administration of such substances as chemotherapy drugs, blood products, antibiotics and even nutrition.[4]

Bone Marrow Transplantation (BMT)

BMT is an aggressive form of treatment that is used for many of the haematological malignancies including the acute and chronic leukaemias, lymphomas, Hodgkin's disease, multiple myeloma, as well as selected solid tumours.[5] The disease free survival for patients after BMT varies based on the type of malignancy, the age of the recipient, and the overall condition of the patient before transplant.[5]

Contrary to the name of this treatment, it is not a surgical procedure. The marrow can be taken from the patient, usually collected during remission (*autologous transplant*), a twin (*syngeneic*), a matched, related donor such as a sibling (*allogeneic*), or matched but unrelated donor (*MUD*).[2,18] This process is known as *harvesting*.[2,37] When the bone marrow is taken from the patient there is the increased risk of contamination with the abnormal or cancerous cells. However, it is now possible to remove, or at least reduce, the numbers of leukaemic cells (a process known as *purging*) or concentrating the necessary stem cells (a process known as *positive selection*).[2] This is done to reduce the risk of relapse.[5,18] The cells are processed, cryopreserved, and stored until the patient has received the conditioning treatment (which can include chemotherapy and radiation).[37]

A very important aspect of ensuring a successful BMT is to match the marrow of the patient and the donor. For a transplantation to have the greatest chance of success, the major transplantation antigens of both donor and host must be matched.[3] These antigens are termed *human leukocyte antigens* (*HLA*).[3,18] Six HLA gene products are typed in preparation for BMT and a full match is termed a 'six out of six' match.[3] Genetic factors determine the match, which are passed on from both parents, and so, the most likely match (one in four) will be with a sibling.[2] Only one-third of patients requiring a BMT will have an HLA-identical sibling.[7] For patients where there is no HLA-matched sibling donor, there are two other solutions. One is to identify an unrelated but closely HLA-matched person willing to donate bone marrow, and the other is to use marrow from a related donor who is less than perfectly matched.[2] Throughout the world there are volunteer registers, called Bone Marrow Donor Registry, making matched, but unrelated (MUD) donors possible.[3] The probability of finding an HLA-identical unrelated match is influenced by race.[7] Also, recently there has been the experimental use of donor marrow that has had the T-cells removed. The T-cells are the mediators of Graft-versus-host Disease (GVHD) and the removal of these cells is seen as ameliorating the severe manifestations of the disease often seen in patients receiving transplants from unrelated donors that are not closely matched.[2] However, the removal of T-cells also seems to lead to increased rates of graft rejection and relapse in patients with leukaemia.[2] Autologous transplants are the most common form of transplant done today.[18] Because the marrow obtained from the patient is perfectly matched, there is no risk of GVHD.[18]

Patients are given high doses of chemotherapy (HDC), and some have total body irradiation (TBI) to destroy all of the malignant cells in the body.[2] These interventions are given to provide a sufficient degree of immunosuppression to avoid the destruction of the donor marrow by the residual cells in the patient; to destroy any remaining residual cancer cells; and in some patients to provide room in the marrow for the cells to grow.[2] The TBI and HDC are administered at doses that are the maximum that can be tolerated.[5] This is called *conditioning* and its purpose is to prepare the body to receive the marrow transplant.[5] Unfortunately, such treatment also destroys many of the normal cells in the body causing side effects that at times need skilled nursing care.[37] Side effects that can be experienced include hair loss, sore mouth or mouth ulcers, nausea, vomiting and diarrhoea.[37] Also, during the period following the HDC and TBI typically all of the patient's blood cells will be severely suppressed and so the patient does not have a defence system for fighting infection (known as *immunocompromised*).[37]

The patient's immune system is immediately rescued by the replacement of the bone marrow.[37] The marrow cells, which have been kept frozen are thawed on the day of the transplant and re-infused into the blood stream where they then make their way to the bone marrow.[5,10] They home to the bony cavities and settle there, regenerating the marrow.[18] The infusion process usually is without incident and quite anticlimactic.[5] Nausea, chest tightness, and chills are not uncommon reactions and usually are limited to the time of infusion.[5,37] Until the time that the individual's immune system begins to function the patient needs total supportive care involving the administration of anti-fungals and antibiotics to protect against infection, reverse isolation, low microbial diet, and blood transfusions to stop haemorrhage and anaemia.[5,10]

The last phase of the transplantation is the engraftment and recovery phase.[37] Evidence that the bone marrow is starting to function with the new marrow is known as *engraftment*.[37] During this time the patient's white cell counts return to normal and the side effects of the conditioning regimen and neutropenia begin to resolve.[37] This process varies widely, lasting from several weeks to months or years.[37]

One of the significant difficulties for BMT is the possibility of rejection.[2] Perhaps the most serious outcome of BMT is when the stem cells do not repopulate and hence do not stimulate the production of new blood cells. The risk of such failure is highest where the 'match' between patient and donor is poor. *Graft rejection* represents destruction of the graft by the immune cells of the host.[2]

The name *Graft-versus-host Disease* (*GVHD*) is given to the condition associated with allogeneic transplantation of the donor's marrow reacting with the recipient's cells.[2,18] The disease is characterised by the donor cells identifying the patient's host cells as foreign and attacking the patient's cells.[5,18] Immediate symptoms of

GVHD, known as the *acute disease,* include skin rashes, diarrhoea, or changes in the liver function causing conditions of jaundice.[2] Continuous GVHD (called *chronic*) can also occur at any time beyond three months and it may affect the skin, mouth, liver, gut and eyes.[2] Strategy to ward against this occurrence is to ensure that the donor's marrow is a match with the patient.[2] Without treatment the condition can be quickly fatal, and so, if problems occur drugs are administered (such as *prednisone, cyclosporine, thalidomide* or *methotrexate*).[2]

The same immune cells that cause GVHD can also attack any of the patient's leukaemia cells. This is a beneficial effect called *graft vs leukaemia effect.*[18]

Other complications with treatment can include pulmonary complications (such as *interstitial pneumonia*), and liver problems (such as *veno-occlusive disease of the liver* which can lead to liver and sometimes kidney failure).[2] Opportunistic infections, with unusual organisms such as *Aspergillus, Cryptococcus* and *Pneumocystis*, are frequent despite preventative measures.[4]

Patients are discharged from the hospital when the blood counts indicate that the graft has taken and they are able to function at home.

Peripheral Blood Stem Cell Transplants (PBSCT)

The potential advantages of collection of cells for PBSCT as compared to BMT include no need for anaesthesia or multiple marrow punctures during donation, and more rapid and reproducible recovery of blood counts after transplantation.[10]

This is similar to BMT but the cells are *harvested* from the blood.[37] There are small numbers of stem cells circulating in the blood (known as *peripheral blood stem cells, PBSC*).[37] Patients can have their own cells collected or can have the cells collected from a related or unrelated donor. Peripheral blood stem cells are harvested through the use of central or peripheral veins and separated by a process called apheresis.[37] The cells are collected in large numbers by running the donor's blood through a *cell separator machine* that separates off the stem cells and returns the blood again to the donor.[8] This process is usually completed in outpatients over a number of hours.[8] Although there are usually insufficient numbers of *PBSCs* circulating in the blood, it is now possible to administer special substances called *growth factors* (*granulocyte colony-stimulating factor/G-CSF* or *granulocyte-macrophage colony-stimulating factor/GM-CSF*) prior to collection to help stimulate (*mobilise*) the production of cells circulating and thus increase the yield.[8]

Umbilical Cord Blood Transplants (UCBT)

Recently it has been recognised that the stem cells remaining in the cord blood of the new born baby after delivery may have potential use for transplantation. The umbilical cord blood contains quite high numbers of stem cells (*haematopoietic progenitor cells*) from the baby.[3] These cells can reconstitute a child's system for producing blood cells (*haematopoietic system*) to provide a self-renewing, perpetual source of all differentiated blood cells.[7] In addition to providing a rich content of stem cells, placental blood provokes a less severe immune response in the recipient than bone marrow.[7] One of the greatest potential clinical advantages of UCBT is that the incidence of GVHD will be lower than expected after MUD.[3] The cells are collected from the discarded cord, causing no harm either to the mother or the baby.[3]

Acknowledging the Harshness

Transplantation has provided quite genuine advances in the treatment of haematological malignancies. Unfortunately, it is not a user friendly medical intervention and patients pay a high cost for the benefits they receive. This hardship is acknowledged in the medical literature. In fact, E. Donnell Thomas, the Nobel Prize winner for his work in BMT, is reported as saying that he hoped the future would bring better ways to treat cancer because transplantation is not a friendly therapy to go through, it is only the best answer presently available.[10]

Appendix 3

WHAT DOES THAT TERM MEAN?

The 'foreign language' of a treating hospital can be overwhelming and daunting to most newcomers. Following is a list of many of the more common terms that are used, accompanied by an explanatory note of the term, which can be used as a quick reference to assist with deciphering the 'talk' of haematology. The terms are alphabetically listed for ease of reference.

- *Acute* – A stage characterised by a rapid progression of the disease requiring immediate treatment.[15]
- *Acute emesis* – is the most common form of chemotherapy-related nausea and vomiting. The onset may take place minutes after the medication is administered, but usually occurs 2-6 hours after administration. It usually lasts up to 24 hours after administration.[25]
- *Adjuvant* – 'Back up' treatment with chemotherapy or radiotherapy following an apparently curative resection of tumour.[16]
- *Aetiology* – Refers to the causes of disease such as infections, radiations, viruses or toxic agents.[18]
- *Alkylating agents* – A class of chemotherapy drugs that interfere with the cell's ability to reproduce.[16,18]
- *Allogeneic Bone Marrow Transplantation* – Involves the transfer of marrow from a donor to another person.[2]
- *Alopecia* – Hair loss.[16]
- *Anaemia* – Depletion of red cells which carry oxygen to the body causing tiredness, dizziness, headaches, and irritability.[17,20]
- *Anaesthesia* – A procedure in which a patient receives medication that blocks out pain.[20]
- *Anaesthesiologist* – A doctor who specialises in the study and administration of anesthesia.[19]

- *Angiography* – Radiological imaging of blood vessels.[26]
- *Anorexia* – Absence or loss of appetite for food.[20]
- *Anticipatory nausea* – A nausea response to any sight, sound, taste, or odour related to treatment. It is believed these responses are conditioned or learned.[25]
- *Asymptomatic* – Without symptoms.[19]
- *Anticoagulation* – Prevention of blood clotting.[26]
- *Anti-emetics* – Medicines used to prevent or relieve nausea and vomiting. Examples of such drugs are Metoclopramide (Maxolon), Ondanestron, Zofran.[20]
- *Antigen* – A substance, foreign to the body, that stimulates the production of antibodies by the immune system. Antigens include foreign proteins, bacteria, viruses, pollen and other materials.[20]
- *Antilymphocyte globulin* – A protein preparation used to treat and prevent graft-versus-host disease.[20]
- *Antimetabolites* – Anti-cancer drugs that interfere with the cell's ability to grow and divide by the cell's ability to produce DNA. Examples include Methotrexate, Mercaptopurine, Fluorouracil, Cytosine Arabinoside.[16,18]
- *Aplasia* – Reduction in the counts of certain blood cells that can be measured in the blood.[26]
- *Aplastic Anaemia* – A condition in which the marrow has degenerated into scar tissue and hence produces too few blood cells.[18]
- *Apoptosis* – Programmed cell death or the mechanism by which chemotherapy and irradiation cause tumour cells to die.[16,18]
- *Aspiration cytology* – A needle is pushed into the marrow and a few drops of fluid are extracted and smeared on a microscope slide. The smear is stained and examined to identify the type of cells.[12]
- *Autologous transplantation* – Involves the use of the patient's own marrow in transplantation. In this form of transplantation there is no risk of GVHD.[2,18]
- *B cells* – White cells (lymphocytes) that make antibodies that destroy foreign substances.[19]
- *Basophil* – Type of granulocyte (white cell) that plays a special

role in allergic reactions and helps in the healing of inflammations.[19]

- *Benign* – Non-cancerous. These cells overproliferate, but unlike malignant cancer cells, they do not invade or metastasise.[18]
- *Biopsy* – A medical procedure involving the removal of a sample of tissue to examine under a microscope to help with the diagnosis of a disease condition. With regards to the bone marrow it is usually a small cylindrical core of bone together with bone marrow about the length of a fingernail and the width of thin spaghetti. It is collected with a specially designed marrow coring needle.[12,20,26]
- *Blasts* – The earliest recognisable forms of all the different types of blood cells.[12]
- *Blast Crisis* – A stage in the development of the *chronic* leukaemias where the disease becomes aggressive and produces large numbers of immature cells.[15]
- *Blood* – A vital organ that supplies food, oxygen, hormones, and other chemicals to all of the body's cells. It helps remove waste products and assists the lymph system in fighting infection.[20]
- *Blood-brain barrier* – A network of blood vessels located around the central nervous system with very closely spaced cells that make it difficult for potentially toxic substances – including anti-cancer drugs – to enter the brain and spinal cord.[19]
- *Blood counts* – A combined test to count red cells, white cells, and platelets, together with a measurement of the amount of haemoglobin the blood contains.[12,26]
- *Blood transfusion* – Blood taken from a donor, prevented from clotting, checked and tested, cross-matched, and administered into the veins of a recipient.[12]
- *Blood type* – Identification of the proteins in a person's blood cells so that transfusions can be given with compatible blood products. Examples of blood types are A+, A-, B+, B-, AB+, O+, O-.[19]
- *Bone Marrow* – The spongy interior of the long bones.[20]
- *Bone Marrow Aspiration* – A process in which a sample of fluid and cells is withdrawn from the bone marrow using a hollow needle.[19]

- *Bone Marrow Transplant* – The transplant procedure begins with the patient or donor providing stem cells. These blood-forming cells are stored while the patient's malignant cells are killed. The stem cells are then returned to the patient to speed the recovery of bone marrow.[18]
- *Brachytherapy* – Treatment with radiation applied at or very near the surface of the body.[20]
- *Burkitt's Lymphoma* – A rare type of aggressive non-Hodgkin's Lymphoma involving the abnormal growth of the *B lymphocyte*. It is the commonest childhood tumour in equatorial Africa.[15]
- *Busulphan* – A drug used in the treatment of conditions such as CML.[17]
- *Cancer* – A general term for more than 100 diseases characterised by uncontrolled, abnormal growth of cells that can invade and destroy healthy tissues.[20]
- *Cannula* – A tube which can be inserted into a vein to allow substances to be fed into the blood circulation.[19]
- *Carcinogen* – A substance that can cause cells to become cancerous.[18]
- *Carcinogenesis* – Refers to the development of cancer. Cancer is believed to arise when one of the cells of the human body escapes the normal growth control mechanism and multiplies irregularly and rapidly.[16]
- *Catheter* – A hollow tube inserted into body for giving or removing substances.[16]
- *Central Nervous System* – The brain, spinal cord, and nerves.[19]
- *Central nervous system (CNS) prophylaxis* – Some types of leukaemia can penetrate the coverings of the brain where ordinary chemotherapy often does not reach. This term refers to the treatments specially targeted at these areas, such as injections into the spinal fluid or radiotherapy of the brain, that are given to address this problem in some conditions.[15,16]
- *Cerebrospinal fluid (CSF)* – Fluid that surrounds and bathes the brain and spinal cord and provides a cushion from shocks.[19]
- *Chemotherapy* – The use of drugs to kill malignant cells. It may be given as a single drug or a combination of drugs.

Chemotherapy drugs are used to destroy cancer cells by interfering with their duplication and growth. Unfortunately, these drugs also affect the normal cell and hence the individual will also experience side-effects from the drugs.[18]

- *Chronic* – Patients do not always require treatment in the chronic stage as the cells affected at this stage are more mature and more able to function. Often individuals with chronic leukaemias can go for extended periods of time without the need for any treatment.[12]

- *Clinical trial* – A carefully designed and executed investigation of a drug, drug dosage, combination of drugs, or other method of treating disease. Each trial is designed to answer one or more scientific questions and to find better ways to prevent or treat disease.[19]

- *CMV* – Cytomegalovirus is the most important infectious cause of severe interstitial pneumonia, especially among patients receiving allogeneic marrow transplantations.[15]

- *CNS Leukaemia* – When the leukaemia cells invade the brain and spinal cord.[15]

- *CNS Prophylaxis* – Therapy administered concurrently with systemic chemotherapy to eliminate any cancer cells remaining in the sanctuary of the CNS.[15]

- *Combination chemotherapy* – This refers to the combination of chemotherapy drugs used in treatment. Combination regimens are commonly known by the first letters of the drugs included.[16,25]

- *Combined Modality therapy* – Various mixtures of distinct treatments which can demand the efforts of a wide assortment of specialists including oncologists, surgeons, pathologists and radiologists.[18]

- *Complete blood count (CBC)* – Measure of the numbers of white cells, red cells, and platelets in a cubic millimetre of blood.[19]

- *Complete remission* – When chemotherapy causes the blood and bone marrow to look normal because of the elimination of most of the malignant cells. This does not mean that all malignant cells have been eradicated. Rather it is the elimination of all measurable or evaluable disease.[16]

- *Computed tomography (CT Scan)* – A body scan or a CAT scan is a very sophisticated technology using computers and X-rays to provide a detailed 3-D picture of the internal organs.[18]
- *Consolidation therapy* – This therapy usually follows induction therapy when the disease is no longer visible. Repeated cycles of chemotherapy are given at reduced doses to further decrease the number of diseased cells.[12,15]
- *Cord Blood Transplants* – Haematopoietic stem cells obtained from the placenta and umbilical cord discarded after a baby is born are used in transplant.[18]
- *Corticosteroids (Steroids)* – A category of synthetic hormones used in treatment and help to suppress GVHD.[20]
- *Cyclophosphamide* – A drug used for immunosuppression and destruction of leukaemia cells.[20]
- *Cyclosporin* – A drug used to treat and prevent graft-versus-host disease.[20]
- *Cytogenetics* – The study of the origin, structure, and function of the chromosomes in the blood cells.[20]
- *Cytology* – The science dealing with the composition and functioning of cells.[26]
- *Cytomegalovirus (CMV)* – This is a virus that is harmless in healthy people but causes serious disease in patients who have had their immune system suppressed through technologies such as Bone Marrow Transplantation. It is one of a group of herpes viruses.[15,19]
- *Cytopenia* – A reduction in the number of different bloods cells circulating in the body.[12]
- *Cytosine arabinoside* – Also known as Ara-C, is given by injection in the treatment of leukaemia. The side effects are vomiting and nausea, and the patient needs to drink lots of water to avoid kidney damage.[17]
- *Cytotoxic* – Causing the death of a cell.[19]
- *Daunorubicin* – A drug given by injection into a vein used in the treatment of leukaemia. It has side effects of nausea and vomiting, hair loss, and possible heart damage if used over a long period.[17]

- *Delayed nausea* – Nausea that develops after the first 24 hours following chemotherapy administration.[25]
- *Differentiation* – The process by which cells mature and become specialised.[19]
- *Disseminated disease* – A stage in the disease where the cancer cells spread to other parts of the body away from the original site.[18]
- *Echocardiogram* – A diagnostic test that uses ultrasound to visualise the interior of the heart and determine how effectively it is functioning.[19]
- *Electrocardiogram (ECG)* – A graphic record of the electric current produced by the contraction of the heart.[19]
- *Eosinophil* – A type of white cell that responds to allergic reactions as well as foreign bacteria.[19]
- *Engraftment* – The successful implantation of donor marrow in the patient's marrow cavities.[20]
- *Epstein Barr Virus* – Usually associated with glandular fever, this virus is also linked with Hodgkin's disease.[23]
- *Erythrocytes* – Red cells circulating in the blood that contain haemoglobin which carries oxygen to all tissues of the body.[18,20]
- *Etoposide* – A drug used in treatment given by mouth or injected into the vein, which has the side effects of hair loss, nausea, loss of co-ordination, inflammation of the mouth, shortness of breath and loss of appetite. If the drug leaks into the surrounding tissue it can do tissue damage around the vein (know as *extravasation*).[17]
- *External catheter* – Indwelling catheter in which one end of the tubing is in the heart and the other end of the tubing sticks out through the skin, for example, a Hickman catheter.[19]
- *Extravasation* – The infiltration or leakage of intravenous fluids or drugs into the local tissue surrounding the administration site.[17]
- *Flare reaction* – A raised, red streak along the course of a vein, which may be mistaken for extravasation.[25]
- *Graft* – Tissue taken from one person (donor) and transferred to another person (recipient or host).[20]
- *Graft Rejection* – Represents destruction of the graft by the immune cells of the host.[2]

- *Graft-versus-host Disease* – A condition that may develop after allogeneic bone marrow transplantation in which the transplanted marrow (graft) attacks the patient's (host's) organs.[19]
- *Graft-versus-leukaemia (GVL)* – The new immune cells from the transplant can attack the cancerous leukaemia cells, resulting in a graft versus leukaemia effect and thereby reducing the risk of a relapse.[18]
- *Granulocytes* – White cells (neutrophils) that fight infection, kill bacteria, and remove damaged tissue. During infection these cells rapidly increase in numbers and destroy the invading bacteria or fungi and then return to normal levels again.[12]
- *Granulocyte-macrophage* or *Granulocyte Colony-stimulating Factor (G-M* or *G-CSF)* – Haematopoietic growth factors administered prior to cell collection for transplantation.[24]
- *Granulocytopenia* – Deficiency of granulocytes (neutrophils, basophils, and eosinophils).[25]
- *Growth factors* – Proteins used to stimulate the production of blood cells.[24]
- *Haematology* – The study of factors associated with blood diseases.[15]
- *Haemoglobin* – The pigment in the red blood cells which facilitates the transportation of oxygen around the body.[20]
- *Hairy Cell Leukaemia* – This condition is characterised by the presence of abnormal cells which under the microscope have 'hair-like' projections.[1,13]
- *Haematologist* – Doctor who specialises in the diagnosis and treatment of disorders of blood and blood-forming tissues.[19]
- *Haematocrit* – The measurement of the proportion of cells to plasma in a sample of blood. Sometimes called packed cell volume (PCV).[19]
- *Haemoglobin* – An iron-rich protein found in red blood cells that carries oxygen.[20]
- *Haematopoiesis* – The development of mature blood cells from precursor cells in bone marrow.[20,25]
- *Haemorrhagic cystitis* – Bleeding from the bladder, which can be a side effect of the drug cytoxan.[19]

- *Heparin solution* – An anticoagulant injected into indwelling catheters between uses to prevent clots.[19]
- *Hepatitis* – Inflammation of the liver by virus or toxic origin. Fever and jaundice are usually present, and sometimes the liver is enlarged.[19]
- *Herpes zoster* – A viral infection that produces shingles, painful skin eruptions that follow the underlying routes of nerves inflamed by the virus.[20]
- *Hickman catheter* – An example of an external catheter. It is an indwelling catheter that has one end of the tubing in the heart and the other end outside the body.[19]
- *Histocompatibility* – The state of similarity between tissues of the donor and the recipient.[20]
- *Histology* – The examination of cells and tissue samples through such technologies as chemical analysis or by looking at them under the microscope.[20]
- *HLA Antigens (Human Leucocyte Antigens)* – Proteins on the surface of cells that are important in transplantation and transfusion. For BMTs, the HLSs on white cells of the patient and potential donor are compared. A perfect HLA match occurs only between identical twins.[19]
- *Host* – In bone marrow transplantation, the person who receives the marrow.[19]
- *Hydroxyurea* – A chemotherapy drug which is an analogue of urea, first synthesised 100 years ago which inhibits cell division.[16]
- *Hypercalcaemia* – High levels of calcium (serum calcium) in the blood caused by the breakdown of bone tissue in diseases such as Multiple Myeloma.[21]
- *Immune system* – A complex network of organs, cells and specialised substances distributed throughout the body and defending it from foreign invaders that cause infection or disease.[20]
- *Immunosuppression* – Reduction of the functions of the immune system either by disease or deliberately through drugs to prevent a reaction against donor marrow cells and to prevent graft-versus-host disease.[20]

- *Indolent lymphomas* – Slow growing Lymphomas that are often asymptomatic other than the painless enlargement of the lymph nodes in the neck.[20]
- *Induction therapy* – Treatment that aims to eradicate all leukaemia cells and allow normal cells to re-populate the marrow.[15]
- *Infusion* – Gradually administering medications or blood products into the blood system of the patient over a long period of time.[19]
- *Infusion pump* – A small, computerised device which allows drugs to be given at home through an IV or indwelling catheter.[19]
- *Interferon* – A drug used in the treatment of some haematological disorders.[17]
- *Interstitial Pneumonia* – Inflammation of the lung tissue, often caused by a virus. A respiratory complication associated with BMT which is characterised by fever, and respiratory distress.[2,20]
- *Intrathecal injection* – The injection of drugs into the cerebrolspinal fluid, usually during a lumbar puncture.[17]
- *Intravenous* – The administration of a substance through a vein.[17,26]
- *Intravenous-access line* (IV) – A hollow metal or plastic tube which is inserted into a vein and attached to tubing, allowing various solutions or medicines to be directly infused into the blood.[19]
- *Inverted Y radiotherapy* – This is radiotherapy given to the lower half of the body, for example, in the pelvis or the central part of the abdomen.[1]
- *Irritant* – A medication that may produce pain and inflammation at the administration site, or along the path of the vein by which it is administered.[25]
- *L-asparaginase* – A drug, usually given by injection, used in treatment that selectively restricts the growth of leukaemia cells. It is associated with allergic reactions in adults but is considered to be well tolerated by children.[17]
- *Leucocyte* – General name for white blood cell.

- *Leucopenia* – A reduction in the number of total circulating white blood cells.[19,25]
- *Leucopheresis* – A process where the white blood cells are removed from the blood before it is returned to the patient.
- *Linear accelerator* – A machine that creates and uses high-energy X-rays to treat cancers.[20]
- *Lumbar puncture* – A medical procedure used for diagnosis where a fine needle is inserted into the fluid around the spinal cord at the lower part of the back to obtain a cell sample. It can also be used to administer drugs to treat CNS disease.[20,26]
- *Lymphangiogram* – X-ray studies of the lymph system after injection of a dye.[20]
- *Lymphocytes* – The white cells found in the blood and lymphatic system that help protect the body from invasion by recognising and reacting to the antigens of the invader. There are three types of lymphocytes, B-cells, T-cells and NK (natural killer) cells.[20]
- *Lymphoblastic lymphoma* – A childhood lymphoma most often of T-cell origin.[20]
- *Lymphomas* – Cancers of the immune system, the complex network of specialised organs and cells that defends the body against infection.[20]
- *Maintenance therapy* – This refers to the administration of low dose drugs to further reduce the residual malignant cells that remain. Such therapy usually follows induction and consolidation chemotherapy where the number of diseased cells have been reduced to a minimum. The aim of maintenance therapy is to keep the number of diseased cells at such a level that the disease either retreats or the immune system is able to destroy it.[12,15]
- *Malignant* – Cancerous (see cancer).[20]
- *Marrow* – Part of the bone rich in haematopoietic, or blood forming, stem cells – primitive cells that multiply and metamorphose into the different components of blood.[18]
- *Metastatic Disease* – Where cancer cells travel through the body to a secondary site and implant resulting in a secondary malignancy.[16]
- *Metastatic Lesions* – The spread of the primary tumour to

produce secondary lesions elsewhere in the body.[16]

- *Metastasis* – The spread of cancer to distant sites in the body.[18]
- *Minimal Residual Disease* – Where it is known that there is still a small amount of malignancy left behind.[16]
- *Monocytes* – Make up five to ten per cent of circulating white blood cells and defend the body against bacterial infection.[20]
- *MRI (Magnetic Resonance Imaging) scan* – A technology based on the use of magnetic fields that produces very detailed pictures of the internal organs. MRI is sensitive to differences in chemical composition and fluid content, and so tumours often present a more dramatic, readily comprehensible appearance in these images than in CT.[18]
- *Monocyte* – A type of white blood cells that 'eats' unwanted material.[20]
- *Mucositis* – Inflammation of the mucous membranes in response to cancer therapies. This may affect the mucous membranes that line the oral (mouth), gastro-intestinal, and/or female reproductive cavities.[20,25]
- *Mycosis Fungoides* – A T-cell lymphoma of the skin.[20]
- *Myelosuppression* – The marrow function being restricted in some way.[12]
- *Neutrophil* – White cells that protect the body by engulfing and ingesting bacteria and other infectious material that enters the body.[12]
- *Neutropenia* – A reduction in white cells known as neutrophils, usually by the drugs given in chemotherapy, which has the consequence of leaving the patient vulnerable to infection.[12,16]
- *NK (Natural Killer) cells* – White cells which kill invading infectious agents, or assist the body's immune system in attacking invading organisms.[21]
- *Oncologist* – A doctor who specialises in treating cancer patients.[18]
- *Oral* – Administered by mouth.[17]
- *Paediatrician* – Doctor who specialises in the care and development of children and the treatment of their diseases.[19]
- *Palliative* – Treatment given to improve symptoms, quality of life,

and possibly to increase life expectancy without prospect of cure.[16]

- *Pancreatitis* – Inflammation of the pancreas which can cause extreme pain, vomiting, hiccoughing, constipation, and collapse.[19]
- *Pancytopenia* – A reduction in all types of blood cells.[12]
- *Partial Response (PR)* – Greater than or equal to 50 per cent reduction in measurable or evaluable disease in the absence of progression in any particular disease site.[16]
- *Pathologist* – Doctor who specialises in examining tissue and diagnosing disease.[19]
- *Peripheral blood stem cell transplant* – Transplantation with peripheral blood stem cells rather than marrow. The cells can be collected from the veins.[24]
- *Petechiae* – An indication of low platelet count seen by small spots of red or purple found on the skin. The spots are actually a form of small haemorrhages.[12]
- *Philadelphia Chromosome* – Discovered in the 1960s, the presence of this abnormal chromosome is important diagnostically in conditions such as CML and ALL.[13]
- *Plasma* – The liquid part of the lymph and the blood.[19]
- *Platelets* – Cells that circulate in the blood to prevent bleeding and help with clotting.[18,20]
- *Ports (Implantable subcutaneous ports)* – Such as Mediport, Infusaport, Port-a-cath, PAS Port, are metal or plastic encased ports with rubber septums attached to a silicone catheter that is inserted into a central vein. These ports are surgically implanted under the skin.[17]
- *Positive Selection* – The concentrated selection of stem cells during the process of collection for transplantation.[2]
- *Prednisolone* – A drug from the family of steroids, given by mouth, used for killing cancer cells in leukaemia treatment. Long term effects can include weight gain, red face, bone weakening, high blood pressure and diabetes. Short courses of these drugs are given in order to avoid these problems.[12]
- *Progenitor cell (Precursor Cell)* – The young cell produced by the bone marrow which will later differentiate into a mature cell.[20]

- *Prognosis* – Expected or probable outcome.[19]
- *Progressive Disease (PD)* – Greater than 25 per cent increase in measurable or evaluable disease or development of a new lesion.[16]
- *Progression Free Survival* – Duration of response to treatment where no measurable increase in tumour size is seen.[16]
- *Prolymphocytic Leukaemia* – This is a rare form of CLL which occurs in the elderly. The abnormal cells in this condition are called pro-lymphocytes. Treatment usually involves chemotherapy and irradiation of the spleen.[1]
- *Prophylaxis* – An attempt to prevent disease.[19]
- *Protocol* – The treatment schedule. It outlines the drugs that will be taken, when they will be taken, and in what dosages. Also includes the dates for procedures (e.g. bone marrow aspiration schedule).[19]
- *Purging* – The process of removing contaminating cancer cells from the cells collected for transplantation.[2]
- *Purpura* – A condition where a severe reduction in platelets leads to purple spots on the skin, often accompanied by bleeding gums.[12]
- *RAD* – Short term for 'radiation absorbed dose' which refers to the amount of radiation absorbed by tissues.[20]
- *Radiologist* – Doctor who specialises in using radiation and radioactive isotopes to diagnose and treat disease.[19]
- *Radiotherapy* – The use of high-dose X-rays or other high-energy rays to kill the malignant cells and shrinks tumours.[16]
- *Regimen* – The combination of drugs and the treatment program for their administration to the patient.[18]
- *Relapse* – This refers to the time that the disease may come back even though it has previously gone into remission. Re-treatment may or may not produce another complete remission.[12,16]
- *Remission* – The time when the disease has been eliminated so that none can be measured clinically, radiologically or on blood tests following treatment.[16]
- *Remission induction* – The initial treatment aimed at eliminating the clinically detectable cancer.[12]

- *Resistance* – Like bacteria resistant to antibiotics, some tumours are able to survive the anti-cancer drugs used to treat them. Certain tumours prove to be drug resistant from the outset, whereas others develop resistance with repeated treatment.[18]
- *Right atrial catheter* – Indwelling catheter with tubing that extends into the heart which provides access for drawing blood and injecting medication.[19]
- *Sanctuary sites* – Sites in the body where the chemotherapy does not reach and hence are likely to harbour disease, for example the testicles or the brain.[16]
- *Secondary Malignancy* – The risk of patients developing a second primary tumour years later is due to the irreversible genetic damage caused by some chemotherapies.[16]
- *Sepsis* – Infectious disease caused by micro-organisms which affects the entire body and is not limited to only one or a few organs or body structures. It is an extremely serious condition.[26]
- *Septicaemia* – A bacterial infection in the blood stream.
- *Side effect* – Unintentional or undesirable secondary effect of treatment.[19]
- *Stable Disease* – Less than 50 per cent decrease or less than 25 per cent increase in measurable or evaluable disease.[16]
- *Staging* – A classification system, using clinical, radiological and surgical techniques, indicating how far the cancer has spread throughout the body.[16]
- *Stem cells* – The single type of precursor cell that eventually produces the different types of blood cells. Although some stem cells circulate in the blood, they reside primarily in the marrow, where they generate a soup of developing blood cells.[18]
- *Stem cell transplantation* – (See Peripheral Blood Stem Cell Transplantation). A form of transplantation used to replace the marrow destroyed by high dose chemotherapy by either the patient's own stem cells collected from their blood stream or bone marrow, or from that of their donor stem cells.[24]
- *Stomatitis* – An inflammatory response affecting the oral cavity or throat.

- *Subcutaneous injection* – An injection into tissue under the skin.[19]
- *Subcutaneous port* – Type of indwelling catheter comprised of a portal under the skin of the chest attached to tubing leading into the heart.[19]
- *Syngeneic transplantation* – Involves transfer of marrow from an identical twin.[2,18]
- *Systemic* – Spread throughout the body, usually via the blood stream. In relation to chemotherapy, the systemic administration of drugs is the distribution of cytotoxics via the blood circulatory system.[18]
- *TBI (Total Body Irradiation)* – Radiation given to all major parts of the body prior to treatments such as BMT with the purpose of eliminating any evidence of cancer cells.[20]
- *T-cells* – Stem cells that develop in the thymus that attacks infected cells, foreign tissue, and cancer cells.[20]
- *Therapeutic* – Pertaining to treatment.[20]
- *Thrombocytes* – Platelets.[19]
- *Thrombocytopenia* – A shortage of platelets which leads to problems with bleeding.[12,16]
- *Topical* – Cream or solution placed on skin.[25]
- *Tumour* – A growth that results from a process when cells stop dividing in their normal orderly way and start to divide in an uncontrolled way.[18]
- *Ultrasound Scan* – An ultrasound examination provides pictures from the echo patterns of soundwaves bounced back from internal organs.[20]
- *Vancomycin* – Antibiotic commonly used to treat infections in indwelling catheters.[19]
- *Vesicants* – Those drugs that have the potential to cause cellular damage when they infiltrate the subcutaneous tissue. Even a minute amount can cause damage, so special precautions must be taken when administering these agents. Examples include, Daunorubicin, Vincristine.[17,25]
- *Vinca Alkaloids* – Chemotherapy drug that interferes with cell division.[16]

- *Vincristine* – A drug used in chemotherapy with leukaemia (ALL) given by injection into a vein. Repeated use can have the short-term side effect of 'pins and needles' and numbing in the fingers and toes, hair thinning or constipation.[16]
- *Vital signs* – Term that describes a patient's pulse, rate of breathing, and blood pressure.[19]
- *Xerostoma* – A dryness of the oral mucosa, the result of decreased production of saliva. This may cause alterations in taste, difficulty in chewing or swallowing, and poor fit of dentures.[25]
- *X-ray* – A type of radiation that can be used at low levels to diagnose disease or in its high-energy form to treat cancer.[20]

Blood Parameters[17]

(Normal blood values may vary slightly with different laboratories).

Haematocrit	Men: 47% (40%–54%) Women: 42% (37%–47%)	
Haemoglobin	Men: 14–18 gm Women: 12–16 gm Children 12–14 gm	
Erythrocytes	Men: $(4.5–6) \times 10^6\,mm^3$ Women: $(4.3–5.5) \times 10^6\,mm^3$	
Reticulocytes	Men: 0.8%–2.5% Women: 0.8%–4.1%	
Leukocytes, total	5,000–10,000 mm^3	100%
• Segmented neutrophils	1,800–6,500 mm^3	40%–60%
• Lymphocytes	1,000–4,000 mm^3	20%–40%
• Monocytes	200–800 mm^3	4%–8%
• Band neutrophils	0–700 mm^3	3%
• Eosinophils	50–400 mm^3	1–3%
• Basophils	0–150 mm^3	0–1%
• Myelocytes	-0-	0%
Platelets		150,000–350,000 mm^3

Appendix 4

REFERENCE LIST

1. Souhami, R. & Tobias, J., (1995) *Cancer and its Management,* Second Edition, Blackwell Science, Cambridge, Massachusetts.
2. Armitage, J., (1994) "Bone Marrow Transplantation", *The New England Journal of Medicine,* 330,12:827–38.
3. Kline, R. & Bertolone, S., (1998) "Umbilical Cord Blood Transplantation: Providing a Donor for Everyone Needing a Bone Marrow Transplant?", *Southern Medical Journal,* 91,9:821–28.
4. Jones, L., (1996) "Progress in Treating Leukaemia", *The Practitioner,* 240:80–6.
5. Johns, A., (1998) "Overview of Bone Marrow and Stem Cell Transplantation", *Journal of Intravenous Nursing,* 21,6: 356–360.
6. Greaves, M., (1993) "Stem Cell Origins of Leukaemia and Curability", *British Journal of Cancer,* 67:413–23.
7. Eder, A. & Jefferies, L., (1998) "A Primer on Placental Blood Banking", *Medical Laboratory Observer,* 30,10:22–32.
8. Atkinson, K., Dodds, A., Milliken, S., Concannon, A., Fay, K., Harris, M., et al., (1995) "Autologous Blood Stem Cell Transplantation for Haematological Malignancy: Treatment–related Mortality of 2%", *Australia and New Zealand Journal of Medicine,* 25: 483–89.
9. Burnett, A. & Eden, O., (1997) "The Treatment of Acute Leukaemia", *Lancet,* 349: 270–75.
10. Owen, P., Connaghan, G., Holland, K. & Steis, R., (1998) "Bone Marrow Transplantation: Cancer Therapy Comes of Age", *The Journal of the Medical Association of Georgia,* 87: 145–48.

11. de Vries, J., (1994) *Cancer and Leukaemia, An Alternative Approach,* Mainstream Publishing Company, Edinburgh.
12. Lilleyman, J., (1994) *Childhood Leukaemia, The Facts,* Oxford University Press, Oxford.
13. Wiernik, P., Canellos, G., Kyle, R., Schiffer, C., (eds). (1991), *Neoplastic Diseases of the Blood,* 2nd Edition, Churchill Livingstone, Inc., New York.
14. Brunning, R. & McKenna, R., (1994) *Atlas of Tumor Pathology: Tumors of the Bone Marrow,* Armed Forces Institute of Pathology, Washington, D.C.
15. DeVita, V., Hellman, S., Rosenberg, S., (eds.), (1997) *Cancer: Principles and Practice of Oncology,* 5th Edition, Lippincott–Raven Publishers, Philadelphia.
16. Barr, L., Cowan, R. & Nicolson, M., (1997) *Churchill's Pocketbook of Oncology,* Churchill Livingstone, NewYork.
17. Preston, F. & Wilfinger, C., (1997) *Memory Bank for Chemotherapy,* Jones and Bartlett Publishers, Boston.
18. Scientific American, *What You Need to Know About Cancer,* WH Freeman and Company, New York.
19. Keene, N., (1999) *Childhood Leukaemia: A Guide for Families & Caregivers,* O'Reilly, Cambridge.
20. Bair, F., (Ed.), (1992) *Cancer Sourcebook,* Health Reference Series Volume 1, Omnigraphics, Inc, Detroit, MI.
21. Horwich, A., (ed.), (1995) *Oncology: A Multidisciplinary Textbook,* Chapman & Hall, London.
22. Haskell, C., (ed)., (1990) *Cancer Treatment,* WB Saunders Company, London.
23. Campbell, K., (1995) The Causes and Incidence of Haematological Malignancies, *Nursing Times,* 91,31:25–28.
24. Donnall, T., (1999) Bone Marrow Transplantation: A Review, *Seminars in Hematology,* 36,4:95–103.
25. Tenenbaum, L., (1994) *Cancer Chemotherapy and Biotherapy: A Reference Guide,* W B Saunders Company, Philadelphia.
26. Heim, M. & Vehling–Kaiser, U., (1994) The Leukaemia Patient as a Partner in Therapy, Volume 2, *Supportive Measures in Oncology,* Jehn, U. & Berghof, H., (eds.), Thieme Medical

Publishers, New York.

27. Holland, J., Frei, E., Bast, R., Kuffe, D., Morton, d., Weichsel-baum, R., (1993) *Cancer Medicine,* 3rd Edition, Volume 2, Lea and Febiger, Philadelphia.

28. Pitot, H., (1986) *Fundamentals of Oncology,* 3rd Edition, Marcel Dekker Inc., New York.

29. Segen, J., (1995) *Current Med Talk: A Dictionary of Medical Terms, Slang and Jargon,* Simon and Schuster, Conneticut.

30. *Webster Medical Desk Dictionary*, (1986) Merriam–Webster Inc., Springield, Massachusetts, USA.

31. Glanze, W., (ed.), *Mosby Dictionary: Medical, Nursing and Allied Health,* 3rd Edition, The C V Mosby Company, Philadelphia.

32. Hoffbrand, A., Pettit, J., (1987) *Clinical Haematology Illustrated,* Churchill Livingstone, London.

33. Chanarin, I., Brozovic, M., Tidmarsh, E. & Waters, D., (1980) *Blood and Its Diseases,* Churchill Livingstone, London.

34. Greaves, M., (1993) Stem Cell Origins of Leukaemia and Curability, *British Journal of Cancer,* 67:413–423.

35. Rice, M., (1994) Progress in Childhood Cancer: Can It Be Maintained?, *The Medical Journal of Australia,* 160:326–331.

36. Kadota, R., (1984) Bone Marrow Transplantation for Diseases of Childhood, *Mayo Clinical Proceedings,* 59:171–184.

37. Johns, A., (1998) Overview of Bone Marrow and Stem Cell Transplantation, *Journal of Intravenous Nursing,* 21,6: 356–360.

Appendix 5

ORGANISATIONS TO CONTACT

Leukaemia Foundation of Australia

Web Address: http://www.leukaemia.com/

Postal Address:
PO Box 222
Fortitude Valley Qld 4006

Telephone: (07) 3250 0500
Fax: (07) 3250 0555

Support Services – Leukaemia Foundation of Queensland
ESA Village
64 Raymond Terrace
South Brisbane Qld 4101
Telephone: (07) 3840 3840
Fax: (07) 3844 7811

Support Services – Leukaemia Foundation of New South Wales
Ground Floor – 44 Harbour Street
Mosman NSW 2088
Telephone: (02) 9969 1762
Fax: (02) 9969 8542
Toll Free: 1 800 620 420
E–mail: leukaemia@ozemail.com.au

Support Services – Leukaemia Foundation South Australia
7 Tucker Street
ADELAIDE SA 5000
Telephone: (08) 8232 9377
Fax: (08) 8232 9311

Support Services – North Queensland
Suite 3/175 Sturt Street
Townsville Qld 4810
Telephone: (07) 4772 5445
Fax: (07) 4772 4756

Support Services – Leukaemia Foundation Victoria
Level 8/535 Bourke Street
Melbourne VIC 3000
Telephone: (03) 9620 1815
Fax: (03) 9620 1422
E–mail: leukvic@leukaemia.com

Support Services – Leukaemia Foundation of Western Australia
11 Freedman Road
MENORA WA 6050
Telephone: (08) 9389 5100
Fax: (08) 9272 9050

Children's Leukaemia and Cancer Society

11 Bamston Terrace
Herston Qld 4006
Telephone: (07) 3252 4719
Fax: (07) 3852 2350
E–mail: clcs@powerup.com.au

Canteen
Web Page: www.canteen.com.au

National Office
Suite 703
Level 7
King York House
32 York Street
Sydney NSW 2000

Postal Address:
GPO Box 3821
Sydney NSW 1044
Telephone: (02) 9262 1022
Fax: (02) 92996322
Toll Free: 1800 639 614

NSW Division (02) 9382 1563
Illawarra Branch (02) 4227 6481
Hunter Branch (02) 4957 6614
Victorian Division (03) 9329 5288
Queensland Division (07) 3252 5188
SA Division (08) 8204 7488
WA Division (08) 9328 2748
Tasmanian Division (03) 6223 7550
ACT Division (02) 6244 4094

The Cancer Patients Assistance Society
C/– Jean Colvin Hospital
Loftus Street
Darling Point
NSW 2027
Telephone: (02) 9362 3429

Make–A–Wish Foundation of Australia
National Registered Office
90 Auburn Road
Hawthorn Vic 3122
Telephone: (Toll Free) 1800 032 260
Fax: (03) 9819 9853

Camp Quality

14 Taylor Street
West Pennant Hills
NSW 2125
Telephone: (02) 9871 0055
Fax: (02) 9871 0239
E–mail: campquality@compuserve.com

Australian Cancer Societies

ACT Cancer Society
159 Maribyrnong Avenue
KALEEN ACT 2617
Tel: (02) 6262 2222
Fax: (02) 6262 2223
E–mail: actcancer@cancer.org.au
Website: www.cancer.org.au

Anti–Cancer Council of Victoria

1 Rathdowne Street
CARLTON SOUTH VIC 3053
Telephone: (03) 9635 5000
Fax: (03) 9635 5270
E–mail: enquiries@accv.org.au
Website: www.accv.org.au

Anti–Cancer Foundation of South Australia

202 Greenhill Road
EASTWOOD SA 5063
Tel: (08) 8291 4111
Fax: (08) 8291 4122
E–mail: act@acf.org.au

Cancer Foundation of Western Australia

334 Rokeby Road
SUBIACO
WA 6008
Telephone: (09) 381 4515

NSW State Cancer Council

153 Dowling Street
WOOLLOOMOOLOO NSW 2011
Tel: (02) 9334 1900
Fax: (02) 9358 1452
E–mail: feedback@nswcc.org.au
Website: www.nswcc.org.au

Cancer Council of the Northern Territory

Shop 3 Casi House
Van Derlyn Drive
CASUARINA NT 0810
Tel: (08) 8927 4888
Fax: (08) 8927 4990
E–mail: uvstop@cancernt.org.au

Queensland Cancer Fund

553 Gregory Terrace
Fortitude Valley QLD 4006
Tel: (07) 3258 2200
Fax: (07) 3257 1306
Telephone: (Toll Free) 1300 361 366
E-mail: qldcf@qldcancer.com.au
Web Site: www.qldcancer.com.au/

Cancer Council of Tasmania

140 Bathurst Street
HOBART TAS 7000
Tel: (03) 6233 2030
Fax: (03) 6233 2123
E-mail: Iride@courier.tas.gov.au
Website: www.tased.edu.au/tasonline/cancer/

Cancer Foundation of Western Australia

334 Rokeby Road
SUBIACO WA 6008
Tel: (08) 9381 4515
Fax: (08) 9381 4523
E-mail: cancerwa@cancerwa.asn.au
Website: www.cancerwa.asn.au